Beyond Stammering

The McGuire Programme for Getting Good
at the Sport of Speaking

Dave McGuire

Souvenir Press

The McGuire Program, California LLC
Email: davemcguire@msn.com
Web site: www.mcguireprogramme.com
Copyright no. TXu 804 545
United States Library of Congress

New Edition October 2002

First published Britain 2003 by
Souvenir Press Ltd,
43 Great Russell Street, London WClB 3PD

Revised edition 2008

ISBN 978 02856 36736

Graphics by Martin O'Brien

Printed in Great Britain by Antony Rowe Ltd, Chippenham, Wiltshire

This book is dedicated to my children, my parents and all those who participated in our mission to help people who stammer throughout the world.

About myself and the programme

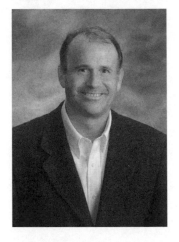 In 1969, after trying several forms of therapy, I had a chance to defeat my severe stammer with the help of Dr Joe Sheehan. At the time he was a psychology professor at UCLA and considered to be one of the very best stammering therapists in the world. His programme was based on active non-avoidance and acceptance of oneself as a stammerer. Although my speech had improved and I was able to develop a career in adolescent psychology, my lack of discipline and downright laziness resulted in many severe relapses that devastated my personal and professional life. In critical moments when I really needed to speak well, the words would not come.

In November 1993, after twenty-four more wasted years, I was given another chance in a diaphragm training programme developed by a famous opera singer in Amsterdam. I found that the diaphragm training resulted in a strong, immediate fluency but would not hold up over time. By applying Dr Sheehan's concepts, however, I found I was able to recover from relapses. Although I am not yet 'permanently' cured, I am totally fluent 99.9 per cent of the time.

I figured the combination of diaphragm training and non-avoidance/role-conflict resolution would be a powerful combination to help many others overcome the affliction of stammering. In February 1994, the McGuire Programme became a reality. In 1995 the programme evolved from 'my' to 'ours' as more graduates have become coaches organising courses and providing critical follow-up support throughout the United Kingdom, Ireland, U.S.A., Norway and Australia.

Dave McGuire

Contents

Preface

by John Harrison

My first encounter with Dave McGuire and the McGuire Programme took place at the Fourth International Conference for People who Stammer, held in Linköping, Sweden, during the summer of 1995. As we chatted about common interests, I learned that Dave had previously run an innovative programme for teenage boys with behavioural problems. Back in the 1960s I had been an active sponsor of a similar kind of residential programme for drug addicts. Both of us had seen that the only way to effect lasting behavioural change was to address the entire person.

Dave's approach to stammering combines his training in psychology with other stammering therapies and sports psychology. Into the mix also went the know-how gained from his experience of working with difficult teenagers. This eclectic background accounts, in part, for the uniqueness of the McGuire Programme. It's also sets Dave apart from most others working in the field of stammering remediation.

At the end of our initial conversation, Dave asked whether I would like to stop by and observe a demonstration of his programme run with several of his graduates. I would indeed, and off we went to his workshop. My first impression of the workshop is still etched in memory – a group of men and women in a circle taking deep breaths with belts strapped around their chests. What in the world were they doing? I wasn't sure what to make of it, but I was really curious. During further conversations at the conference, it became clear that Dave and I shared a common view of stammering, and we promised to stay in touch once the conference was over.

I was intrigued with the McGuire Programme. As someone who had stammered for roughly 30 years and who had made a full and lasting recovery, I saw a recovery strategy similar to what I, myself, had followed. As an émigré to California from New York in the early 1960s, I had immersed myself in the personal growth movement that was flourishing on America's west coast. I'd grown up with a very fuzzy image of myself and needed to change many beliefs and behaviours that did not serve me well. In working to build self-esteem and get my own house in order, something very interesting happened: my stammering gradually slipped away.

According to most speech therapists, this was not supposed to happen. The prevailing belief was 'once a stammerer, always a stammerer'. But that was evidently not true, at least for some people. Over time, I saw that my stammering was not simply a product of bad speech behaviours, it was also a reflection of who I was as an individual – how I thought and felt, how I functioned, what I believed. My speech blocks had everything to do with the system of self that I had created, a system that supported a dysfluent way of speaking. Therefore, to make permanent changes in my speech, I had to address a total system that included my emotions, perceptions, beliefs, intentions, and speech behaviours. And it all had to be brought into alignment.

What so intrigued me about the McGuire Programme was that this was the first programme I'd encountered that took a broad, holistic approach to stammering and that touched on many of the same issues that I had addressed in my own recovery. Not only did the McGuire Method focus on the speech process itself, it also focused on the underlying factors that supported the stammering behaviour. Even today, several characteristics of the programme are truly unusual.

- The programme uses costal breathing to keep the breath open and prevent speech blocks. The programme focuses not just on 'can I speak?' but on 'how do I want to speak?' Eloquence is a stop on the path to fluency.
- Graduates do the teaching and coaching – there is no professional staff of speech therapists – giving teeth to the concepts that (1) the real experts are those who have personally worked through the problem, and (2) best way to learn something is to teach it to others.
- McGuire also has the best long-term follow-up programme in the world. It is free and open ended. Coaches and those being

coached routinely connect by phone and email and those connections often reach half way around the world.

- A graduate can go through the programme any number of times for just a very small token fee.
- Graduates are free to suggest changes to the course, which accounts for the fact that the McGuire Programme continues to evolve.

This book will be useful to anyone who wants to gain a clear and detailed picture of what is involved in the recovery process. As you'll discover, the road will take you through more than just changes in how to speak and how to manage speech blocks. It will help bring to awareness the subtle ways in which you've shaped your world to support your stammering. You'll also acquire a better sense of those issues that need to be addressed in order to break through into a newer, freer way of speaking.

You'll learn, not just about how to acquire fluency, but how to *keep* it. You'll develop an understanding of the various factors that trigger relapses – why they happen, and what to do about them.

The text is full of sports analogies – highly appropriate, consid-
ering that speaking, like tennis, is a performance skill and subject to many of the same pressures and pitfalls. You'll be introduced to various practice techniques needed to etch new speech behaviours into your psyche, and you'll be offered various recovery strategies that you can fall back on when you run into turbulence and slip into relapse.

Finally, you'll gain a perspective on the 'life games' that can either undermine or support your recovery from stammering.

Can you recover from stammering just by reading this book? That's like asking, 'Can you get from London to Bath by simply reading a roadmap?' In both cases, the answer is 'not likely'. If you want to get from point A to point B, you need to put yourself in motion, commit yourself to the journey, and decide you won't quit until you reach your destination. Some people have the discipline to make the trip themselves. Others will want assistance, either from a speech therapist, or by enrolling in one of the trainings presented by the McGuire programme in various countries. But whatever your choice, this book is an excellent 'map' that will help you proceed on your journey better informed and with a clearer set of objectives.

Since I995, I have been privileged to meet many McGuire graduates, and I have observed several four-day trainings in their entirety. I've heard the graduates' stories. I've seen the results. What is clear is that recovering from stammering is, for most, a difficult and challenging trip. It requires persistence, a clear commitment, a strong sense of dedication, and a willingness to step outside your comfort zone repeatedly.

But given a hearty resolve, it is also clear that the programme works. I invite you to open your mind and allow yourself to discover a total approach to the age-old problem of chronic stammering.

J.H

2003

John C. Harrison is no stranger to the problems of stammering. He showed a marked disfluency at the age of three, and two years later underwent therapy at the National Hospital for Speech and Hearing Disorders in New York City. But this and later efforts at therapy during his school years were not successful and he struggled with stammering throughout college and well into adulthood.

Harrison's involvement in a broad variety of personal growth programmes over three decades has given him a unique insight into the nature and dynamics of the stammering person. Today, he is fully recovered and no longer deals with a stammering problem.

One of the earliest members of the National Stuttering Association, Harrison was an eighteen-year member of the Board of Directors and is currently the editor of the NSA's monthly newsletter Letting Go. Harrison has run workshops for the stammering and the professional communities across the U.S. and Canada as well as in Ireland, the U.K., and Australia. He has been published in *Advance Magazine* and the *Journal of Fluency Disorders* and has presented at conventions of the American Speech Language Hearing Association and the California Speech Language Hearing Association, as well as at the First World Congress on Fluency Disorders in Munich, Germany. Harrison lives with his wife, Doris, a graphic designer, in San Francisco where he works as a freelance writer.

Introduction

This book started out in 1994 as the manual for a world-wide programme known as 'The McGuire Programme,™ Freedom's Road®'. It is an association of regional programmes owned and instructed by people who are in the process of going from people who stammer uncontrollably, to people who enjoy speaking and do it well. Our mission is to help other people who stammer throughout the world.

Two years after the millennium, I was approached by Souvenir Press to make this available to the public. So here it is . . . but with some cautions:

This book is not for those who are satisfied with the constraints dictated by stammering. Nor is it for those looking for a permanent cure. We cannot guarantee that you will never stammer again any more than any tennis camp could guarantee Pete Sampras that he will never again double fault. It is a way, if you're willing to work hard and be courageous, to become a good, even eloquent speaker, and have fun playing this wonderful sport of verbal communication.

You should also know that this will indeed be very much like learning a skilled sport such as tennis or skiing from a book. If you're talented and persistent with a good work ethic, you can probably make significant progress. Chances are, however, you would need help from a qualified tennis/ski instructor. Same with the sport of speaking. Although some people can make significant improvements in their speech through this book, most will need personal instruction.

If you try this on your own, give it six months of your best effort. If there is significant progress, then keep going. If your gut tells you this is the right path, you've sincerely done your best, but you are not happy with the progress, it probably means that you need coaching and follow-up support. Contact us, then, through our website: www.mcguireprogramme.com and apply to join our programme.

If you've given this a fair shot, but don't think it is the right approach for you, try something else. There are many programmes and many good therapists for those who stammer. But do keep trying.

PART ONE:

How to get it

*Most of the important things in the world
have been accomplished by people
who have kept on trying
when there seemed
to be no hope at all.*
DALE CARNEGIE

'Getting it' is like any other significant accomplishment. You
are better off having goals and objectives.

OUR GOAL: Eloquence . . . *'Playing to win'*

Ultimately, your goal is to become a strong, eloquent
speaker rather than simply a 'non-stammerer'. As in sports
psychology this requires developing the mentality of 'playing
to win' rather than 'playing not to lose'. To achieve this, we
have the following objectives:

Physically: the objective is to speak powerfully from the thorax by
retraining your costal diaphragm.

Mentally: there are six objectives:
• to understand the dynamics of stammering
• to counteract the tendency to 'hold-back' and use avoidance

mechanisms
- to deal with the fear through concentration and non-avoidance techniques
- to accept yourself as a recovering stammerer until you have proven yourself 'a fluent speaker with occasional reminders of your past affliction'
- to develop an assertive attitude to attack your remaining feared situations
- to understand the process of relapse and how to counteract it

Emotionally: once you have dealt with the fear, the objective is to let go and *have fun* speaking.

Spiritually: the objective is self-actualisation. Once your verbal self is set free, who will be doing the talking? Are you the person you want to be? This positive internal change – beliefs, intentions, perceptions, etc. – is necessary to hold on to your fluency.

CHAPTER ONE:

Understanding the mental and emotional part of stammering

'Kangaroo in the Headlights'

Before we can start to do something about your stammer, we need to have a base of understanding of at least one theory of what it's all about. This chapter is about the mental and emotional part. The next chapter will get into the physical part. Then, in the third chapter, you'll get what you need to become a good speaker.

Volumes of high falutin stuff have been written about stammering, the cause of which has not been proven. Some says it's genetic. Others say it's the result of a neurological defect. Others say it's purely psychological. Nothing has been proved scientifically. For purposes of doing something about it, our belief is that it follows the dynamics of behaviour and sports psychology, and results in physical dysfunctions that, in turn, intensify the psychological one, and ends up in a vicious cycle.

By 'psychology', we mean the mental, emotional and attitudinal factors involved. For the most part it is the same thing that musicians and athletes go through when they are afraid to make a mistake. It's called:

'Choking'

You can see it as 'performance fear' gone wild. You see it during penalty kicks at important soccer matches. It's relatively easy for a good player to make a goal from that distance even against the best of goalies. But how many times have you soccer fans seen the ball sail high or wide? And you *know* that what is going on in the player's head is 'better not blow it!'

Or the tennis player who blows the easy shot or double faults away a point that would win the match or get him or her back in the game. Or the trumpet player who blows the high note during a performance. Or the field goal kicker in American Football blowing a point he can make with his eyes closed in practice. Or O'Neil missing an important free throw.

For us who stammer, it is the fear of stammering – of blowing getting out that word.

'Kangaroo in the headlights': The multi approach-avoidance conflict

One Australian graduate of our programme came up with this one to explain how he felt during a stammering block. Kangaroo starts across the road, sees the car/headlights coming, can't decide whether to keep going across the road, or go back. So he freezes in the road.

It best describes a dynamic, which comes from some very basic experiments in behaviourist psychology, mostly BF Skinner, where rats were put in cages with food at one end. But there was a catch. There was also an electric grid, so that every time the rats tried to get the food, they were given electric shocks. The rats wanted the food, but were afraid of the shock. This came to be known as the 'single approach-avoidance conflict'.

Now, take those same rats and put another food and shock at the other end of the box. Here you have a double approach-avoidance conflict. Put other lanes in the cage with the same reward and punishment at each end, and you have a 'multiple approach-avoidance

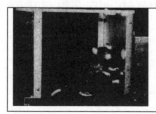

To do two things at once is to do neither.
Publilius Syrus

conflict'. The more lanes, the more stressed the rats become. Sort of like that kangaroo getting caught in the headlights in a busy intersection.

Same with people. The more unresolved choices, the higher the stress. It could be argued that the more unresolved conflicts we have, the more dysfunctional we are. Perhaps mental health simply boils down to how quickly and effectively we can resolve our approach-avoidance conflicts.

How does this apply to stammering? In a single approach avoidance conflict, the desire for food is *the desire to be perceived as fluent.* The fear of an electric shock is *the fear of being perceived as a stammerer.* But, with those who stammer, it is seldom a single approach-avoidance conflict. Those conflicts, which we share with fluent speakers, become turbo charged by our stammering. Here are a few of the biggies:

The fear of being too slow versus desire to communicate quickly: This goes back to childhood. One problem with stammering is that it takes more time to speak. Especially with children, many people don't want to wait and will be obvious with their impatience.

Fear of disrespect versus desire for respect: This applies to when you are dealing with someone whose perceived social status is higher than yours. But not always. It can apply to teenagers and children – anyone from whom you want respect. It is difficult to get this respect as an out-of-control stammer.

Fear of being perceived as incompetent versus desire to be perceived as competent: In business or formal social situations, you want the other people to see you as competent in whatever you are doing. When dealing with a nasty block while trying to explain something to customers, colleagues, etc. some folks will perceive you as incompetent. And, of course, you blow this up in your own mind.

Fear of not speaking versus desire to shut up: Sometimes you don't want to speak to anyone. You want to be left alone. Then

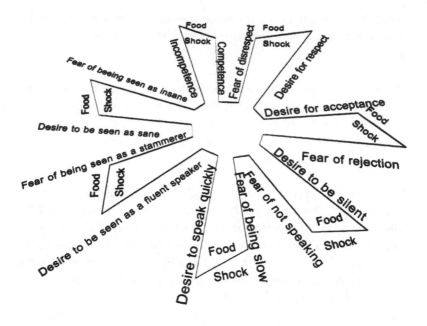

The more approach-avoidance conflicts, the more severe the stammer

some bored nerd bursts into your office wanting to chat. Or your sister-in-law comes over right before your Sunday afternoon nap. You don't want to communicate, but you're afraid not to.

Fear of being perceived as insane versus desire to be perceived as sane: A stammerer using lots of tricks and avoidances no longer looks like a stammerer. People understand stammering. They don't understand jaw chomping, leg slapping, tongue thrusts, and head jerking. Some folks will see it as crazy. Very few people want to be perceived as insane.

Fear of rejection versus desire for acceptance: Almost every one wants social acceptance. Almost nobody wants to be rejected. Especially with potential love relationships.

The more approach-avoidance conflicts, the more severe the stammer.

Not your usual fear-based choking

The pattern is the same, but there are some notable differences between performance fear-based choking of sports and music, and that of stammering. Although one can cite many examples of young athletes and musicians being bullied by parents and coaches for failure, the humiliation and trauma experienced by a person (especially the young) who stammers is infinitely more intense and the psychological damage more severe. An athlete or musician does not need to do the sport or music to feel part of the human race. But the person who stammers can't do a very basic, necessary function that very young kids can do so easily. There is a huge difference between Johnny who can't make a free throw in basketball, and Teddy who stands there in front of the class trying for five minutes to get through a simple sentence.

Then, there is the dynamic that sometimes, on a cursed 'good day', even the worst person who stammers can be quite fluent. Problem is the people around him are thinking, 'there! See! He *can* do it. Just has to put his mind to it and stop being lazy.' Then the next day comes, things are going bad, words won't come regardless of the struggle and number of tricks being used, and those around the young person who stammers give the message covertly or overtly of: 'What's the matter with you!? You were talking perfectly yesterday.' Pressure to perform increases.

Young athletes who have been abused have the option of 'getting out of Dodge' at some point. In other words, they can stop playing their sport or musical instrument when they are at an age to stand up to adults and make their own decisions. Not so with stammering people. We can't dump our racquets or trombone into the garbage and walk away. We *have* to speak (and speak reasonably well) to prosper in society. We *have* to play this sport.

The cycle of panic

It can be argued that most psychological things tend to run in cycles. With stammering it can best be described as a Cycle of Panic. Not just fear. Panic.

Starting with:

Performance fear. This is tied into fear of failure, which specifically is tied to the fear of stammering, or, more precisely, the fear of being seen as a person who stammers, it leads to:

Confusion. You don't know where to go, what to do. It's like walking though a minefield not knowing if you'll get blown up with your next step. By adding this confusion to the fear, you started getting into the realm of panic, which leads to:

Holding back: Someone going through a minefield not knowing where the mines are will hold back on taking that next step, or inch their way through. When this fear of stepping on a mine becomes great enough, everything freezes up and the person is caught in the:

Approach-avoidance conflict: Or the mental block. If, for the person who stammers, there is no escape or resolution, the experience is a 'physical block'. All those muscles, especially the diaphragm, that are necessary to perform this sport of speaking freeze. The delivery of the word, just like the flubbed extra point kick, is blown and the person who stammers experiences: **Shame, self-hate, guilt:** But a very intense version. Because we cannot stop speaking, us people who stammer develop various mechanisms and struggles to avoid the act of stammering by substituting words, slapping legs, biting tongues, etc. Although these might get out the feared word part way through the minefield of the speaking situation, the act of avoiding (running away), which often makes the struggling stammer seem bizarre, increasing the original performance fear.

Unless a miracle happens, this cycle repeats itself, becoming more intense each time (increasing the severity of that mish-mash of blocking, struggle and avoidance called 'stammering') until the situation ends.

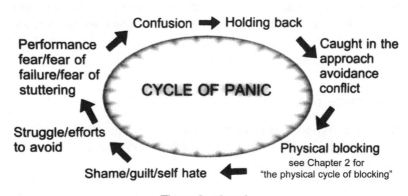

Confusion ➡ Holding back

Performance fear/fear of failure/fear of stuttering

Caught in the approach avoidance conflict

CYCLE OF PANIC

Struggle/efforts to avoid

Shame/guilt/self hate ⬅

Physical blocking
see Chapter 2 for
"the physical cycle of blocking"

The cycle of panic

But that's not the end of it. The memory of this sticks around for the next difficult speaking situation where it raises it's not-so-pretty head, taps you on the shoulder and whispers in your ear 'remember what happened the last time . . .'.

Roots of the fear

My personal recollection of as a severely stammering young junior high school student standing before a class of Victorville street thugs enduring their merciless teasing while trying to deliver the dreaded 'oral report' – and the hours or days leading up to it – was that death would have been much preferable. I've often wondered, why the fear of stammering is so overwhelming. Why is it so important to speak clearly? What's so bad about stammering?

Being different: Breaking it down, the simple answer is that it makes us different. But in a negative way. We're different because we are seen as incompetent. After all, speaking (reasonably well) is so easy. Little kids can do it without even thinking, like walking down the street. We are seen as incompetent because sometimes we can speak fluently. Just when the pressure is on that we fall apart. It's like someone who needs crutches to walk suddenly being able to run and dance and play tennis, then, just because something upset him, can't take two steps without the crutches. Now we've added a major mental weakness or even insanity to what was perceived as a 'physical' problem.

Need for perfection: Let's face it. The more perfect we are in this society, the more goodies we get. So the desire to be good looking, look young, have a great body, be intelligent and educated, be rich, have a big house and impressive cars, etc. is overwhelming. You hear from pop psychologists that we need to love and accept ourselves and others regardless of the faults, but the reality is still we are judged by what we *do* and how well we do it. We shouldn't 'be' what we do, but the reality is that we are indeed 'are' what we do.

Factor into this not being able to do that very basic thing called 'talking', and the fear of not being perfect versus the desire to be perfect is very strong.

Alone: It would appear that for at least thousands of years, we survived as herd creatures. A predator, if it meant to do harm to one member, would have to deal with the whole mob. To be 'different' meant risking rejection from the tribe or clan. Such rejection meant the possibility of being cast out into the wilderness alone without the protection of the herd.

Then you have the very basic need to find a mate and procreate. Unless being different led to being an innovative leader or, say, inventing something new and useful to the clan, those who did not measure up to the normal standards found it very hard to find a mate. Probably truer for males than for females when it came/comes to stammering.

Figure we evolved for generations with this fear of rejection and being alone and not 'qualifying' for a mate. Apply it to a young person struggling *alone* through an oral report in class and you get the picture.

One of the most effective things about the McGuire programme is the support system. We learned early on that even the best technique or method is ineffective without support from others with the same goal that addresses this fear of being alone. (In my own recovery, yes even as the founder of the programme and author of this book, I have run into difficult times with my usually strong speech. It never ceases to amaze me the dramatic improvement that comes when one of my former students gives a bit of support).

Persecution: Add to this such practices as branding or cutting out pieces of the tongues of people who stammer in the Middle Ages that might very well go back for millennia. If Carl Jung's theories of the 'collective human consciousness' or even the theories of reincarnation that such trauma gets passed on from generation to generation is valid, you have another deep seated source of panic and terror.

Covert and overt stammering

There are two types of people who stammer: One type is very successful at hiding the stammer by skilful use of tricks and word substitution and situation avoidance. We refer to these folks as 'coverts'. Many times those whom he or she has known for years do not know that s/he stammers. But for a successful covert person who stammers, it means going through life waiting for the axe to fall . . . waiting for that situation where s/he can't get out of the situation or there just isn't another word to substitute for the word that s/he knows will cause a big embarrassing block.

In many ways, a covert person who stammers will have a tougher time in treatment because it is relatively easy to go back to tricks and avoidance that have kept up the facade of normal speaking.

Someone who is an overt stammerer is simply an-unsuccessful covert stammerer. S/he tries to avoid and use tricks, but the struggle and blocking is there for everyone to see. Perhaps s/he was successful for a while at hiding the stammer, but ran into a few too many unavoidable, untrickable, inescapable words and situations which caused him or her to lose confidence in their hiding/avoiding strategies and panic started to rule the day. Coverts can control the panic; overts can't.

Generally, the worse the stammer, or more overt, the better. Things can only get better. You tend to get much support from those around you when improvement is starting to be observable. You're not faced with the daunting task of the covert person who stammers of explaining to friends, associates, (and sometimes family) that you do indeed have a stuttering problem which is the first foundational step of *any* good stammering treatment programme.

For more insight into covert stammering, read 'Battling' by the Irish graduate and instructor, Patrick Merrigan, in the last section of this book.

"You are what you resist"

An instructor from Scotland, Allan McGroarty, uses this statement on courses he instructs. It is very true for those who stammer. All the struggle that you see on the surface of an overt person who stammers and under the surface of a covert person who stammers is fuelled by efforts not to stammer. The more you resist being a person who stammers, the more you maintain the identity of a person who stammers.

'Then why try to become a fluent speaker?' you will ask. There is a big difference between trying not to stammer, and trying to speak well. In sports psychology, it's the difference between playing to win and playing not to lose. It's a matter of mental focus. Someone trying not to lose a tennis match, or not to stammer, is focusing on those things that cause poor performance. Someone 'playing to win', or trying to be an effective, eloquent speaker, is focusing on those things that improve performance.

CHAPTER TWO:

The physical factor

Breathing, articulators, vocal cords

> *Nothing in life is to be feared.*
> *It is only to be understood.*
> MARIE CURIE (1867–1934)

Whether you buy our belief in the psychology of stammering, or someone else's, its manifestation is some kind of physical behaviour. Something less than productive happens to those muscles that produce the spoken word as a result of the approach-avoidance conflicts, cycle of panic, and avoidance mechanisms.

Enough research has been done to verify that the physical dynamics of a stammering block involves dysfunctions of breathing, the vocal cords, and/or articulators. Of these, we believe the most significant contributor to and possibly the physical precipitator of the stammering block – and the least attended to in most other therapies – is breathing. The main organ responsible for this dysfunction is a muscle called the diaphragm.

Some basic breathing anatomy

Let's start with the torso, which is all that area above the hips and below the neck. Your torso is divided into two chambers: the abdomen, that area below the diaphragm, and above the hip; and the thorax, which is the area above the diaphragm below the neck also

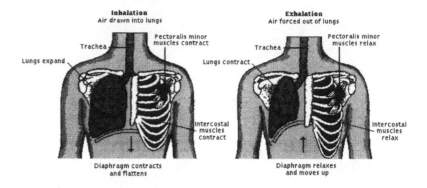

Anatomy of breathing

known as the chest. Actually, there are three chambers because the thorax is divided into two separate breathing chambers.

These two breathing chambers that house the lungs are actually vacuum chambers. The main mechanism for operating these vacuum chambers is the diaphragm, which also divides the thorax from the abdomen.

When it's time to take a breath of air, the brain sends a message to the diaphragm to contract. When the diaphragm contracts, it becomes smaller and the top, called the 'central tendon' moves towards the abdomen. This creates more space in the chest cavities, which creates a vacuum. Just like pulling the plunger out on a bicycle pump. Air rushes in and fills the little air sacks (alveoli) in the lungs.

When it's time to breath out or speak, the diaphragm relaxes therefore becoming bigger and moving deeper into the thorax. This means less space in the thorax. Less space means less vacuum. Less vacuum means the air goes out of the lungs.

The diaphragm

Now that you have the big picture of the breathing mechanism, let's talk about the diaphragm itself. It is shaped like a huge bell in the thorax. The heart sits right in the middle and is attached to the diaphragm by the same membrane that lines the torso. Under the left lobe of the diaphragm is the stomach. Under the right lobe is the liver.

The diaphragm is one of the biggest muscles in the body, and *the* biggest semi-automatic muscle in the body. Semi-automatic means that it operates much like your eyelashes – part of its function you have no conscious control over, part you do have conscious control over. This is mainly so that you can keep on breathing while you're asleep. It is also so that you can do other things than having to think constantly: 'Okay, now, on the count of three, breathe in, breathe out, breathe in, breathe out' all day long. That would be almost as bad as having to think consciously about flipping television channels.

All muscles are to a certain extent involuntary. Just watch what you do the next time someone yells at you unexpectedly. Or the next time you are walking down the street and someone sets off a bomb in the bar across the street. Your arms fly up to cover your face, or your chest, or your groin. What are your muscles doing? They are contracting. They are preparing to protect, or to fight, or to run away. And, of course, you also inhale sharply.

Now why do you suppose you would inhale sharply? Well, it is because your diaphragm is a muscle. Like all muscles, it tends to contract as a response to fear. Unfortunately, the diaphragm needs to relax in order to speak. You have two powerful forces trying to move the diaphragm in opposite directions. You have the natural response to fear contracting the diaphragm and drawing air in. Then you have your own desire to speak trying to relax the diaphragm so that air can move over the vocal cords. The result is what? A frozen diaphragm, of course. Or a diaphragm, as one researcher found, that is moving chaotically. Frozen, chaotic diaphragm means no airflow or chaotic airflow. No airflow means no speech. Chaotic airflow means . . . well chaotic speech. Both can be a symptom of that phenomenon called stammering.

Home of the soul

The ancient Greeks called the diaphragm 'the home of the soul' because the nerve that controls the diaphragm is called the Phrenic nerve – Phrenic is the Greek word for soul. Homer even referred to it as the home of the emotions. I suspect he was right. Don't know about you, but when I'm angry I feel it in my chest. When I'm crying, there may be tears coming out of my eyes, but the feeling is in my chest. When I laugh, you may hear it from my mouth, but I feel it in my chest. When I'm afraid, I may have sweat running from my face, but I feel it in my chest.

Then the ancient Greeks had a word that sounds like 'exphrenos', which means to speak from the emotions. We would probably translate that today as 'speaking from the heart'.

Assuming for now the diaphragm is the physical centre of our emotions, it becomes more than an ordinary muscle reacting to fear by contracting. It is the muscle where we feel the emotion of fear. Add to this the fact we cannot see the diaphragm functioning, and we begin to see why stammering is such a mysterious affliction.

The two structures of the diaphragm – crural and costal

Before, I referred to the diaphragm as one big muscle that controls breathing by controlling the vacuum in the two chambers of the thorax. In terms of control of the crown (central tendon) of the diaphragm, this is true; however, this crown is controlled by two separate sets of muscles that can function independently. These parts are the 'Crural' and the 'Costal'.

Crural: This structure of the diaphragm is attached to the spine. When it contracts, it displaces your abdomen in order to make room for the vacuum in your thorax to draw in air. This is functioning when your tummy is moving when you breathe. If your chest happens to move up and down, it is a secondary result of the abdomen displacement.

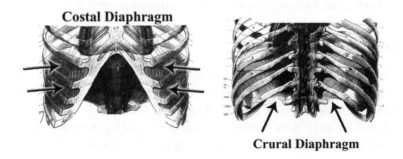

Costal Diaphragm

Crural Diaphragm

Crural and costal diaphragm

The crural diaphragm is responsible for probably 98 per cent of your breathing.

It is what operates when you are sleeping and when your body doesn't need a lot of air. It therefore operates mostly automatically. Most folks speak from air produced by the crural diaphragm.

Costal: Looking at the pictures, you can see that the costal diaphragm is much larger than the crural diaphragm. It is attached to the bottom of the ribs. When the costal diaphragm contracts, the rib cage also pulls up and out expanding the volume of the thorax to create a vacuum. (Whether the costal part of the diaphragm plays a role in pulling the ribs up and out is unknown, but, for sure, you know that the costal diaphragm is being used when the ribs are expanding.)

You know your costal diaphragm is working when you yawn. The body is just asking for more oxygen. It is used during heavy exercise, heavy coughing and sneezing. You also use it sometimes when you shout or sing loudly. Its action is usually voluntary – you have control over when it is used or not used.

In 1962, one of the world's experts on the diaphragm, Dr Peter Macklem of McGill university in Canada, did a study to determine if the various functions of the diaphragm. A dog – whose respiratory function is basically the same as humans – was hooked up to electrodes where the C5, C6 and C7 nerve roots (C3, C4, C5 in humans) could be individually stimulated. All these roots join into the phrenic nerve then branches into two parts above the heart. The right branch goes to the crural part of the diaphragm, and the left into the costal part.

What happened was that when the dog's C7 root was stimulated, only the crural diaphragm contracted. When the C5 was stimulated, only the costal diaphragm contracted and the ribs expanded, which meant there was also some interaction with the intercostal muscles. When the C6 nerve root was stimulated, both parts of the diaphragms contracted and ribs expanded.

So why is this important to you? Well, go back to the description of the crural diaphragm. It is this diaphragm, which controls the airflow for normal speaking. Therefore it is the crural diaphragm, which is chronically contracting in response to fear in those who stammer.

Now, we can retrain the crural diaphragm for years to counteract this chronic contracting during speech. Or we can spend years desensitising ourselves to the fear. Or we can do it quicker by bypassing the crural diaphragm and going to the costal diaphragm and its separate nerves.

Why should you believe that costal diaphragm training can help you become fluent? Because many stammerers who have trained themselves to speak from the costal diaphragm are now fluent. And many, like myself, became fluent very quickly. Not only fluent, but eloquent. Why? Perhaps for two reasons. First, is that you become a more powerful speaker for the same reason an opera singer sings better by using the costal diaphragm. Secondly, if the diaphragm is the home of the emotions, by focusing on this and training yourself to speak from the thorax means you are speaking from your emotions. Which means you are speaking the truth – speaking from the heart. Such speakers are usually eloquent.

The costal diaphragm is a fresh start for stammerers. Not only is there a fresh breathing muscle, there is a fresh breathing nerve – the C3 root and the left branch of the Phrenic nerve.

The ribs, intercostal muscles, alveoli, abdomonus rectus, abdominal obliques, and elastic fibres in the lungs

If you want to know every little detail about the physiological mechanics of inhalation and exhalation, you're in for some work as it is an incredibly complex process. For those who insist on understanding before taking one step further, here is an overview. The rest you can find in any medical book on the respiratory system.

Your ribs act like a bucket handle. Or a pump handle. Their hinges are on the vertebrae. There are many muscles controlling the movement of the ribs including the costal diaphragm, sternocleidomastoids, scapular elevators, anterior serrati, and scaleni erectus muscles of the spine. The main muscles, however, for rib movement are the interior and exterior intercostal muscles. These are very short but stretchable muscles connecting the ribs to each other. (Yes, the next time you're digging into barbecued ribs, the stuff you're enjoying is the poor beast's intercostal muscles.) When the costal diaphragm and the exterior intercostal muscles contract during inhalation, it pulls your ribs up and therefore out. Another set of muscles, the papasternal intercartelaginous, also lift the front of the ribs. The interior intercostal muscles are still relaxed, but get stretched. This increases the area of the thorax and helps to create the vacuum. When the costal diaphragm and intercostal muscles relax during normal exhalation, the ribs return (down and in) to their resting position.

In normal exhalation, the main force of outward airflow is elastic recoil from the little air sacks in the lungs called alveoli. There is also an elastic recoil from other tissues such as elastic fibres in the lung and the pleural membrane. If inhalation was from the costal diaphragm/external intercostals, there is also elastic recoil from the internal intercostal muscles that have been stretched. The rate and smoothness is of normal exhalation is controlled by the relaxation of the crural and/or costal diaphragm and, mainly, the exterior.

Now, if more forced exhalation of air is required, say, for shouting, tuba playing, blowing up balloons etc., the interior intercostals contract to make the ribs collapse faster. Then here comes the big abdominal muscle along with his buddies the external and internal obliques, and transversus abdominis. These contract to make the abdomen smaller thereby forcing the diaphragm domes faster up into the thorax. This apparently functions by way of releasing vacuum pressure in the abdomen and by literally pushing the abdominal contents up against the domes of the diaphragm lobes. The rectus abdominus also helps to collapse the rib cage by pulling downward on it.

The theory

So now that we sort of have the physical idea of stammering in relation to respiratory physiology, let's put it into a usable theory:

*   The diaphragm (probably the crural diaphragm) in 'those who stammer' is chronically contracting when it should be relaxing which disrupts the airflow (also a thing called 'subglottic pressure') causing primary blocking and, later, secondary avoidance and distraction behaviours. This will be elaborated upon below.
*   Different muscles are involved in different types of inhalation, and these determine which respiratory muscles are involved in

expiration and therefore speaking. By inhaling (mainly) from the costal diaphragm and exterior intercostal muscles, it allows the costal diaphragm to be the diaphragm of expiration during speaking.

- The costal diaphragm, with its separate enervation, is not conditioned to contract uncontrollably during speaking. Therefore, using the costal diaphragm in speaking results in increased fluency.
- By engaging the costal diaphragm, the interior intercostals (mainly) are also brought into play during speaking either through elastic recoil or direct contractions or both, which further gives greater control over subglottic pressure and more fluency.

And to restate the second premise: To use the costal diaphragm and interior intercostal muscles as the primary muscles of exhalation, it is necessary to use the costal diaphragm and exterior intercostal muscles as the primary muscles of inspiration. Therefore, again, the muscles of inspiration determine which muscles of expiration are used. Some muscles of expiration contribute to stammering, others contribute to increased fluency.

The physical cycle of blocking

Going back to the Cycle of Panic where the fear of being seen as someone who stammers leads to blocking, guilt/shame/self-hate, avoidance mechanisms then more fear and panic, let's look closer at the physical dynamics of this thing called 'blocking':

Our belief is that the diaphragm is the main physical reason or epicentre of the stammering block. But there are other structures involved, mainly the vocal cords and articulators, that have also become, to varying degrees, dysfunctional in stammering speech. After some observations, it appears to happen according to the following cycle:

1. The crural diaphragm contracts in response to fear resulting in reduced or stopped air flow.
2. This in turn lowers the pressure below the vocal cords (subglottic pressure) to the point where vocal cord vibration is no longer possible as the pressure below the vocal cords needs to be higher than the atmospheric pressure in order to produce sound.
3. The vocal cords, probably in an automatic response to this reduced subglottic pressure, become tighter (closer together) to rebuild the pressure. This, over time, becomes chaotic.

4. As our first concept of speaking has something to do with the lips and tongue (articulators), the habit of struggling and distorting these structures to get out our words becomes habitual and uncontrollable. We have had no idea that perhaps 50 per cent of the physical problem is with the unseen/unfelt diaphragm, and another 25 per cent is with the also unseen/unfelt vocal cords, so most of our attention has been on our articulators that we can see and feel. As developing young stammerer, I remember thinking: 'It got to be something wrong with my mouth 'cause that's what makes the words . . . so if I can just control my mouth I should be able to . . . .' Over control is as bad, if not worse, than undercontrol. So a diagram of this process would look something like:

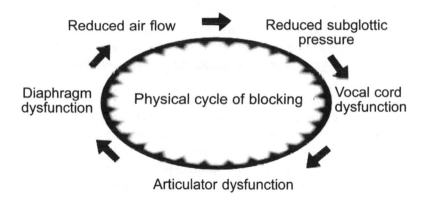

The Physical Cycle of Blocking

So what to do about it? Well, here's an outline of brief answers:
1. For diaphragm dysfunction: training to speak from the Costal Diaphragm.
2. For vocal cord dysfunction: using a deep and breathy tone and the short aggressive hit and hold (hit and hold).
3. For articulator dysfunction: hit and hold/short aggressive hit and hold and keeping the speaking process down in the chest.

Confused? Well, you should be, because all this has yet to be described and explained and elaborated upon in the next chapters. Read on.

CHAPTER THREE:

Developing a new speaking technique

'If not you, who? If not now, when?'
MALCOLM N. (SIXTY-THREE-YEAR-OLD GRADUATE
WHO COMPLETED THE COURSE IN SYDNEY, FEBRUARY, 2000)

Say you're a tennis player and you have this massive double fault-ing problem. You have a reasonably good serve when there's no pressure, but every time you're serving an important point, you blow both your first and second serves. So you go to a teaching pro who, if he or she is worth their salt will first correct any technical faults you may have. This can be anything from a bad ball toss, to a bad grip, to improper stance, to not dropping the racquet head behind your back to no spin on the ball . . . or combinations thereof. Once the technique has been improved and, through hard work, you've 'grooved' the new technical habit to replace the ineffective habit, a good pro will show you some things to deal with the 'fear of double faulting'.

And this is exactly what will happen here. You'll be shown new, more effective speaking techniques to counteract the dysfunction in the diaphragm, articulators and vocal cords. Once you've worked hard and drilled the new techniques into automatic habits, we will show you some things to do to deal with the fear of stammering. In other chapters we'll give you some basic ideas of how to reach your potential and heal the damage that stammering has done to you.

Preparation

So, here we go. First some preparation. Like any serious athlete or musician, you will need to:

Commit: to following our directions for at least six months. Commitment means giving it your best shot. Do your best. If it doesn't work you can always try something else (and give that your honest best shot). But if you're going to do this, then do it.

Give up: your old tricks and avoidance mechanisms that got you by before. These have nothing to do with good speaking technique and will impede your progress. More than that, tricks and avoidance will increase your fear making even the best techniques ineffective.

Resolve to change your speaking personality: I was told by one fine old gentleman that, to overcome stammering, one must 'totally and permanently change one's speaking personality'. He had conquered his own stammer and was very wise. But when you change your speaking personality you are, when you think about it, changing your whole personality – at least that part of your which other people experience. More on this later when we get to psychological strategies.

Work hard: to develop the new physical and mental habits boils down to hard work. If you come to this already with a good work ethic, great. If not, then it's time you developed a good work ethic.

Be disciplined: there are things that you will have to do which you won't necessarily want to do because of whatever combination of excuses you can find. You will need discipline to do what you don't want (but need) to do to reach your goal. If you don't have the personal skill of self-discipline, then resolve to develop it.

Courage: just starting this journey takes courage. You are, or should be, throwing down the gauntlet against your old stammer. You will need courage to keep from using tricks and avoiding words and situations. You will need courage to attack those fears, which have ruled your life and held you back. You will need courage to change. Courage can be developed.

Be kind to yourself: no self-flagellation, putting yourself down, saying nasty things about yourself if you don't get the hang of this right away. Like many of us who stammer, judging yourself too harshly is an ingrained habit. Like any athlete or musician trying to improve, self-flagellation is mega counter-productive. It prevents you from adequately concentrating on the task at hand, keeps you in the past, keeps you from moving forward.

Get a tape recorder and a mirror large enough to see the top half of your body.

If you have a trusted friend who will spend some long hours helping you to learn and drill this, and providing you with a speaking partner, great. True friend indeed. Do nice things for them.

Some new, more effective physical habits

This whole thing is much about developing new physical and mental habits. Here are the physical habits:

Answer to the breathing problem: the Costal Diaphragm

Remember in the last chapter our theory that your crural diaphragm has the nasty habit of reacting to the fear and panic by contracting, thereby shutting off the flow of air over the vocal cords? No airflow, no speech.

Well, we could spend the next thousand or so years retraining your crural diaphragm not to react to the fear. But we won't. We're going to take the fast track and go to that new part of the diaphragm and a different branch of the Phrenic nerve. We're going to learn to breathe from the COSTAL DIAPHRAGM.

> *He who has begun has half done.*
> *Dare to be wise; begin!*
> HORACE (65–8 B.C.)

This will be the hardest part of it all. Do your best:
1. Stand up straight. Would be good to have a full-length mirror.
2. Get a belt. Put it around your chest above the mid-point. Make sure it is tight enough to stay in place after you exhale, but not so tight that it causes pain.
3. Inhale fast and full through your mouth by expanding your ribs.

Make sure you have maximum rib expansion and maximum inhalation. Feel the pressure on the belt. Make sure you are breathing only from the ribs/thorax (costal diaphragm), and not the abdomen (crural diaphragm).

4. Without stopping after the inhale, exhale all your air moderately slowly (again through your mouth). Feel the pressure of the belt around your chest release.
5. Make sure both inhalations and exhalations are smooth and continuous even though inhalation is faster than exhalation.
6. Pause for a minimum of five seconds before you inhale again.

Repeat this pause, inhale/expand, exhale fifty times. Really pay attention that you have it right as it is the foundation for everything else. Look in the mirror to make sure:

1. Your shoulders are down and relaxed especially during the inhale.
2. Your neck is relaxed.
3. Your face is relaxed.
4. Your mouth and throat are open just enough to inhale/exhale quietly.

You may feel tingly and light headed. Don't worry. You are hyperventilating. Just make your pauses longer after the exhale.

You can sit now, but keep your hands on your knees, your feet flat on the ground, and your back straight, preferably away from the back of the chair. Remember that it is not good to sit for too long (bad for your circulation), so alternate standing and sitting.

After about 50 to 100 of these costal breaths, one right after the other (remember to pause), **you must commit to breathing in this manner, taking a costal breath at least twice a minute during your waking hours** except while eating. Probably for the rest of your life. Just remember that people generally breathe too shallow, so developing the habit of deep costal breathing will be good for your health and will relieve a lot of stress.

CAUTION

Do not take these full costal breaths while eating because you risk choking.

Because you are now doing much of your breathing through your mouth, you must drink more fluids to keep your vocal cords from drying.

Nose versus mouth breathing

Although It is important to feel what it is to inhale and exhale through the mouth while you take a fast and full costal breath, and to drill this mouth breathing for the first few days, you need to be aware that the nose is an important filtration system. Therefore, after you the first week, make sure that you:

1. Inhale through the nose when you are not speaking.
2. Inhale though the mouth when you are about to speak and are speaking, as this is necessary to keep down the inhalation noise and to allow more air more quickly.
3. You can choose yourself whether to release residual air through the mouth or nose. Sometimes it is better to release residual air through the nose as then you are not breathing in the listener's face and it lessens the drying effect of releasing through the mouth.
4. If you experience vocal cord problems as a result of inhaling through the mouth, even if you are only doing it while speaking, then start inhaling through the nose even during the speaking process, but be aware that a 'fast and full' costal breath through the nose can be quite noisy.

Dealing with struggle in the articulators: Introduction to 'hit and hold'

From the last chapter, we know that (unless you are a particularly good covert person who stammers), there is much struggle and distortion of those muscles in and around the mouth, including the tongue, that we use to form the words. And it is probably this distortion more than anything that makes us such a target for the bullies. To deal with this, we've developed a technique called the 'hit and hold'. The professionals would refer to this as a 'block modifier'.

Do what you're afraid of doing: So what is it about a feared word that makes it so fearful? For many of us who stammer, it has been the first sound of the feared word. We generally have been afraid to enunciate this first sound fully because we're afraid of getting stuck – either stuck before we've got a sound out, or stuck in the middle of the sound so we can't go on to the next sound. Therefore we've avoided the first sound with soft contact or skipped over the first sound altogether. Or we've used various tricks. Or we've avoided the word completely. Whatever we have done, it has been avoidance behaviour that has absolutely nothing to do with good, articulate speech.

Because we are afraid of approaching this first sound of the feared word, and because we are afraid of getting stuck in the sound, the principles of avoidance reduction say that we have to attack. We are afraid of the first sound, so we attack the first sound. We are afraid of staying in the feared sound, so we purposefully stay in the first sound by holding and prolonging. We are afraid of doing this *so we are doing it* . . .

First, you must realise that all the struggle going- on in the articulators are efforts to avoid the act of stammering and, in the final stages of panic, simply to get the word out. It reinforces hold back, and has become habituated and counterproductive . . . and again, it has nothing to do with good, articulate speech.

(You'll argue, maybe, that hit and hold also has nothing to do with articulate speech, but if you look at it as an exercise like lifting weights to improve athletic performance, you'll see that it is a great tool for improving articulation.)

The idea is to 'hit' that very first sound of a word and hold it out for a second or two without distorting. You have to be fairly aggressive to counteract the habit of holding back and avoiding. And you might have to hold it out longer and stick with it until you can release the sound smoothly. Remember to stick with the sound of the first letter and not to prolong the second letter (usually a vowel). Now, this is a bit tricky, so read closely:

The dreaded 'plosive' consonant sounds:
Those of us who stammer generally have the most trouble with what are known as 'plosive' or 'hard' sounds. These are: B, (hard) C, D, G, K, P, Q, T, so we'll start with these.

When attacking these sounds, realise that they have two sounds: the first pure 'b' sound followed by an 'ah' sound. So the tendency is to hit and hold that second 'b' sound rather than the first so something like 'bingo' will sound like 'baahingo' rather than 'bbb-bingo'. So listen to yourself and use a tape recorder to make sure that first sound of a plosive letter is the first and not the second sound.

So let's use this to apply your new breathing technique, using your tape recorder and mirror, to hit and holding the VERY FIRST sound of the following words. Hold out the H&H for about three seconds to get the feel of it.

Benny, Cattle, David, Gate, Kelly, Peter, Quick, Table. Now, get the dictionary and practise the words beginning with plosive sounds.

Non-plosive consonant sounds:

(Soft) C as in celery, F, (soft) G as in Gerry, H (see below), J, L, M, N, R, S, V, W, X, Y, Z

These are pretty straightforward as there is not the same hidden second sound in each letter. The tricky part you'll find is smooth release. Get your dictionary, and go to work on words starting with these non-plosive consonants, paying particular attention to the release. And again, use your tape recorder and mirror.

The very first sound of the H is difficult to get hold of. The tendency is to blow out all your air before any vibration occurs. So with this sound, and this sound only, go to the second sound, almost always a vowel, that you can vocalise which is generally the second letter. So figure: 'happy = (h)aaaaaappy'.

Vowel sounds:

A, E, I, O, U. These are vocalised in your vocal cords, but not articulated. In a feared situation, the tendency is to 'choke' the word out to get some kind of sound in the vocal cords.

So get out the dictionary, and again with full costal breathing technique, practice on all the vowel sounds until it is comfortable.

Dealing with struggle in the vocal cords: Deep, breathy tone

Struggle and distortion in the vocal cords mainly happen with vowel sounds. You've just learned about hit and holding these, which is the first step in counteracting struggle in both the articulators and vocal cords, but the vocal cords require something special.

The higher the tone of your voice the more strained your vocal cords. Remember, the vocal cords are controlled by muscles, so we need to keep these as relaxed as possible by developing a deep tone.

So give it a try, using everything you've learned before on some words beginning with vowels. Listen to the tone and keep trying to get it as deep as you can. You might want to use a piano and follow the notes down the keyboard until you reach the tone that is as deep as possible, yet comfortable.

Once you've got down deep enough, you need to add some air so that you're getting a breathy sound. The idea of it here is to keep the deep tone from turning 'guttural' thereby straining the vocal cords. By adding a bit of breathiness to the sound you are allowing the vocal cords to stay even more relaxed.

Now, drill all you've learned so far until it feels comfortable. Remember, just one word at a time. When it's feeling good, move on to:

A new way of speaking

We're going to take all you've learned so far and start adding more words per breath still using the Hit and Hold on EVERY word, with a deep and breathy tone. Make up a two to five word phrase. For right now, limit it to five words per breath in this pattern:
More specifically:

- Pause for 5 seconds.
- Take a full and fast costal breath.
- Say your five-word phrase-making, and make sure that there is no gap between the inhale and delivery.
- Release all your air.
- Pause for 5 seconds before repeating the phrase or saying a new phrase.

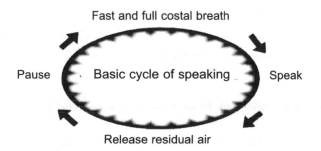

Fast and full costal breath

Pause — Basic cycle of speaking — Speak

Release residual air

The basic cycle of speaking

Hear your words before you say them: auditory imaging

In sports, this is called 'visual imaging'. A tennis player sees the flight of the ball from strings to the exact spot in the opposite court BEFORE hitting the serve or groundstroke. Once the technique is habitualised, this helps the body to perform the action by programming what needs to be done.

In music it is called 'auditory imaging'. When I was having trouble with my attacks and initial intonation, my trombone teacher would instruct me to 'hear', for example, a B flat, before taking a breath to play the actual note. Sure enough, the note came out cleanly (good attack) and in tune (good intonation). My breathing and 'chops' (lips) knew exactly what to do to produce a clean and accurate B flat.

Start with one word. Hear it with your air released. Take a fast, full costal breath. Say the word. Do this about 20 times. When you think you got it, add another word, and another until you are up to, for now, a maximum 5-word phrase.

At this point, you can start speaking without the hit-and-hold, but keep throwing these in now and again for practice. Remember, though, that you need to 'hear' the hit and hold just as accurately as you would a normally articulated word.

Once you've mastered the 'auditory imaging' and feel confident, it's time to add more stuff to the above steps and put it all into what we call 'the checklist'. Much of this will be new, but explanations will follow.

The Checklist

This is the complete method in a nutshell. Following this outline are explanations of the components.

Pause
* Resist time pressure. Imagine being rushed, and wait.
* Make sure your residual air is released. This, in tennis, is the same as starting in the 'ready position' before hitting a groundstoke.
* Centre and clarify. For right now, this just means concentrate, and remember that you are a person who stammers making a

sincere effort to overcome stammering and become a good speaker. There is a whole chapter devoted to more of this.

- Hear what you want to say. Same as above.
- Establish eye contact. It's part of being a good speaker, and looking away is like running away. And running away is avoidance, which increases the fear and lead to panic and blocking. More about this under 'explanations'.

Inhale

- Take a fast costal breath. But not so fast that it becomes shallow and noisy. See detailed explanation later in this chapter.
- Make sure it is a FULL breath. You'll know by how the belt tightens on your chest. See explanation later.
- Make sure your shoulders are down, and face and neck relaxed. Keep it quiet by opening your mouth just wide enough to not make a whistling sound, and open your throat enough so it doesn't make a noise as it passes over your vocal cords. Don't make it obvious you are taking a humongous breath (see explanation).

Speak

- Perfect timing. Make sure there is no gap between the inhale and exhale/delivery. Make especially sure that you aren't throwing in one of those sneaky tricks to help you get out the word (see explanation).
- Make your first sound 'assertive'. Musicians refer to this at the 'attacking the note'. Psychologically, it will counteract the tendency we who stammer have to hold back (explanation forthcoming).
- Feel it resonating in your rib cage and imagine it traveling to a distant spot. Good speaking technique, especially for public speaking, and another way to counteract the holding back that leads to blocking.
- Remember the 'deep and breathy' tone.
- Keep moving forward, no holding back. Once you're off to a good start, keep going until it's time to release your air and pause.
- Articulate. Give each word its proper pronunciation and enunciation. Remember that 'hit and hold' ultimately is to help you develop good articulation.

- Release your residual air. Note that this important step is also at the top.

So that's it. The famous McGuire Programme checklist. As you practise it, think about:

Isolate and exaggerate

A tennis player trying to improve his game will isolate and work on one specific aspect of his technique. A full shoulder turn for more power or a closed racket face for more topspin. While concentrating on one thing, however, other components tend to fall apart. While thinking about a full shoulder turn, for example, he might not get the racquet under the ball thereby sending the ball into the net.

Therefore, a tennis player must practise every component until, like a perfectly tuned engine, everything is smoothly and automatically working together. You must go through your checklist to make sure everything is working smoothly and automatically together.

A tennis player trying to improve his game will also exaggerate as well as focus on every component. If he is working on a shoulder turn, he will turn until he is looking over his shoulder at the ball and has his chin resting on his shoulder. He knows that in a tight match the tension will result in less-than-full shoulder rotation. By exaggerating in practice, however, he is ensuring that his rotation will at least be adequate. Barely adequate rotation during practice will result in an inadequate rotation in a tight competitive match.

Same with your speaking technique. You exaggerate your fast, full inhale/rib expansion during practice so it is adequate in a feared situation. You exaggerate and prolong your hit and hold in practice so that it will hold up under pressure. Same with all the other components.

Additional components

You'll need a few other things to get you going. Practise these as you would anything else.

Block Release
If you feel a block coming, release your air, pause and start again. You can either go back to the start of the phrase or start where you

left off. Do this also if you have a normal dysfluent stumble or want to rephrase. Practise this even if your technique is perfect and you don't feel any blocks.

Cancellation

We are trying to develop a new habit, so if it is not perfect, go back and do it again. We have many many years of reinforcing the old dysfunctional habit of speaking. Remember, every time you let yourself get away with the old way of speaking, especially any kind of struggle, distortion or use of tricks or avoiding certain words or sounds, this becomes stronger. So make sure you pay attention, listen and, when possible in a mirror, look at yourself. If it's not right, do it again.

And, finally . . . .

Concentration

Getting out of your own way.

Tim Gallway, in his *Inner Game of Tennis*, talks about your body already knowing exactly how to produce a good tennis stroke. One simply needs to get one's ego out of the way and concentrate fully on the ball. The book *Zen and the Art of Archery* talks about this too.

After you have spent enough time learning to speak from the diaphragm, concentration will allow all those complicated things to happen automatically. When learning a skill, you must think about what you are doing and struggle at first. But later, thinking gets in your way.

What about your mouth and vocal cords? Even the worst stammerer has periods of fluency. Your mouth and vocal cords have known exactly what to do for many years. It has been the lack of diaphragm control that has needed the attention. Once you have retrained your diaphragm, concentrating on almost anything such as the reflection in your listener's eyes, or the deepness of your voice, or a spot on your thumb allows your body to perform and co-ordinate all those functions necessary for speech.

> *The art of medicine consists of amusing the patient*
> *while nature cures the disease.*
> VOLTAIRE

Fear

Concentration is a great tool for controlling fear and keeping it from turning into panic. We'll be dealing with this more extensively from some different angles in the next chapter.

More explanations

Although I explained much of the 'whys' of what you do, it is good for you to get a more detailed explanation for some of these things. Keep in mind, however, that much understanding will come, many times, from taking action.

> *Explaining metaphysics to the nation –*
> *I wish he would explain his explanation.*
> LORD BYRON (1788–1824)

Why the belt?

The idea is that you need to develop the habit of speaking from the costal diaphragm rather that the crural diaphragm. This means learning to inhale by using your ribs rather than your abdomen. Feeling the belt tighten on your chest lets you know that you are indeed using your ribs to inhale. It also gets your attention down in your chest where your voice is resonating rather than up in your vocal cords and articulators.

Why the checklist?

Funny thing about San Francisco's Golden Gate Bridge. It is constantly being painted. It takes so long to paint the thing that by the time the painters have finished, it is time to start over again. Same with your new speaking personality. You will find that while you are working on, say, formulation your 'fast and full' will suffer. So you go back to fast and full and get that back in shape. And so forth. You keep at it until every part of the method is perfect and running smoothly as a whole system. Unlike the Golden Gate Bridge, you will come to the point you can stop working on it. In this respect, it is more like sanding and polishing a rough piece of wood. Perhaps better is the process of writing and editing a book.

Musicians and athletes experience this. While a novice piano player is focusing on his left hand, his right-hand performance falls apart. He keeps working on it until it is functioning perfectly and automatically. Then he can focus on experiencing the music.

A tennis player will do the same thing. While concentrating on getting his racquet under the ball, his shoulder turn or footwork may fall apart. So he goes back and concentrates on these things for a while. Once his form is perfect and working together smoothly as a system, he can think about the strategy needed to win a match.

Why resist time pressure?

Ever notice a good tennis player before they serve? Good tennis players take a lot of time before they serve. They bounce the ball. They see what part of the service court they want to hit. They centre themselves. If their ball toss is not perfect, they let it go and toss again. Good tennis players give themselves all the time they need to produce a good serve. They do not rush. Bad tennis players usually rush their serves and everything else.

The same thing with speaking. Those of us who stammer almost universally succumb to time pressure. We panic and rush thinking the universe will come to an end if we don't respond immediately. It is one of their many approach-avoidance conflicts. Desire to be quick enough versus fear of being too slow. It's probably the approach-avoidance conflict that started the whole stammering process when you were developing your verbal skills.

By forcing yourself to pause before you speak, you are resolving that conflict which has to do with time. For many of you, it will be the first time you have ever given yourself time before you speak.

'Take your time' has probably been suggested to you before but hasn't helped. It probably made things worse because the fear increased during the pause. It was also giving you the message that there is something terribly wrong with stammering. But now the game has changed. Before, you had no idea of the role of your diaphragm in stammering. All the time in the world will not help a tennis player produce a good serve if he does not have the basic serving technique. All the pausing in the world is not going to help you if your breathing technique is wrong.

The other thing about the resisting time pressure is dignity. Before, anyone could make you rush. Someone rushing is not dignified. So hold your dignity while you pause. Let the other people rush, and be undignified when they speak.

Resisting time pressure is like all the rest – you have to practise it if you expect it to hold up during the big game.

Why release your air?
Your diaphragm has responded to fear by freezing until it is now chronic. The treatment for this is movement – as much movement as possible. By fully exhaling your air, your diaphragm is starting at its maximum 'up' position so it can go down to it's maximum 'down' position, thereby getting a full range of motion.

As a sports analogy, it is like returning to the 'ready' position after hitting a ground-stroke or volley. Or returning to a deep knee-bend after making a turn in skiing. Releasing residual air allows you to be 'ready' for the next speaking phrase.

If you don't release, you will get into a pattern of taking shorter and shorter breaths. This can develop into just another trick just to get the word out. The result is you gasping for air before a feared word – playing not to lose. You should focus on this right before you start to speak, and at the completion of each phrase.

Why centre and clarify?
This is about knowing where you're coming from before you speak. Who are you? What do you want from these words you are about to speak? Is what you're about to say the whole truth? Is it honourable? Are you trying to impress the listener(s)? What are you feeling? If you do not know 'where' your words are coming from, you risk another approach-avoidance conflict.

One of the most important tasks during centring is deciding what role you will assume going into a situation. You will either be a recovering stammerer or a fluent speaker depending on how you have been doing in practice and other situations. If your fear level is high and you have been blocking frequently and/or using tricks and avoiding words, then the role you should assume is that of a recovering stammerer. If, however, you have proved to yourself that you can stay fluent even when feeling fear, you can go ahead and assume the role of a fluent speaker while being willing and comfortable with going back to the role of a recovering stammerer should things get out of control.

Centring has a lot to do with reaching the emotional and self-actualisation goals. Failure to make progress in this area will prevent you from getting and holding eloquent speech. This is covered more in the chapter on centring and clarifying. In addition, you are encouraged to seek out the many resources books and workshops – for personal growth.

Why hear yourself say it before you say it?
Besides what was already mentioned about programming your body, there is a very good chance that, between the fear and avoidance, you seldom or never really think about what you wanted to say before you say it. Most people would do well to think before they speak. Again, remember that just because so many people advised you to do this doesn't mean it's something to be rejected.

In a feared situation the words that best describe you are fearful, panicked, confused. Most of you cannot win a difficult argument under these circumstances. All your opponent has to do is set off your fear, which sets off your confusion. Argument over. A verbal opponent senses this instinctively just as a dog senses fear. Problem is, in today's society, we generally defend ourselves and fight with words.

Formulating your sentence or phrase (saying it to yourself word for word) before you say it also forces you to concentrate. Now, this does not mean that you are editing out the feared words. You can, like any good writer or speaker, edit out unnecessary words, but editing out feared words will destroy your progress.

You may hear the argument that it is good to be spontaneous. Maybe so. Sometimes. But most times, being spontaneous is a good way to keep sticking your foot in your mouth. Especially in business.

> *If one does not know to which port one is sailing,*
> *no wind is favourable.*
> SENECA

Why eye contact?
Those of us who stammer, historically, have poor eye contact. For those of us who stammer, the reason is obvious – we can't bear to see the expression on the listener's face as we struggle to do what

so many people take for granted. Poor eye contact is undignified, a sign of fear or lying, is uncomfortable for our listener, and is not eloquent. Good eye contact is a sign of self-assurance, respect, honesty, and is more comfortable for the listener. Although you do not want to stare during your pause, you must establish eye contact before you begin to speak.

More important, poor eye contact is an act of avoidance. You're avoiding looking at what may be a disrespectful, pitiful, patronising, etc. expression. Remember, do what you're afraid of doing. And by establishing that solid eye contact, you are starting to move forward, which is countering the tendency to 'hold back' that is the psychological foundation of stammering.

For a while, you will need to exaggerate eye contact to make sure you will do it satisfactorily in a feared situation. Later you will expand this to seeing the reflection or pupil in your listener's eye.

> *Father told me that if I ever met a lady in a dress like*
> *yours,*
> *I must look her in the eye.*
> CHARLES, PRINCE OF WALES
>
> (ON SUSAN HAMPSHIRE S DÉCOLLETAGE)

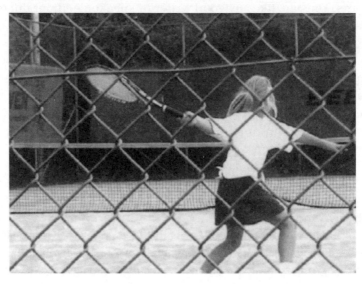

Why a <u>full</u> rib expansion and air intake?

True, you don't really need a full breath of air to speak. But you do need a full costal diaphragm motion to overcome the tendency to freeze in feared situations. A full inhale + rib expansion = full costal diaphragm motion.

In tennis groundstrokes, it is critically important to have a full shoulder and hip turn in preparation to hit the ball. In this way, you can maximum power and control with minimum effort and minimum unforced errors. Let me introduce you to Stephanie. At the time of writing, she's nine years old. She beats boys regularly who are much older. Look at her classic shoulder turn as she prepares to strike the ball. Because her preparation was full, her swing can be full. She has practiced – and exaggerated – this for many hours so that it will at least be adequate under tournament pressure. Now look at her serve. Knees bent. Back arched. Shoulders turned. Everything ready to go up after the ball and deliver a serve with spin, power and accuracy. Same with your rib expansion and inhale.

Why a fast rib expansion and inhalation?

A slow inhalation/rib expansion might be good enough for safe, non-feared situations. But it won't hold up, generally, in tough pressure situations. If it is too slow, it can also be that you are already holding back and trying to avoid.

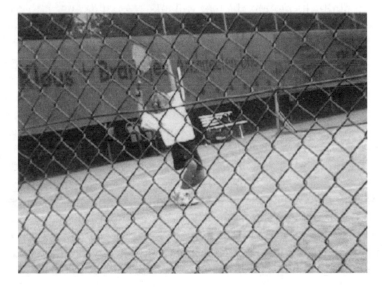

By keeping your costal inhalation fast, you are counteracting the tendency to hold back,. Just be a bit careful that you don't make it so fast that you sacrifice fullness.

To go back to Steph in the above pictures, note that she is prepared in plenty of time both on the forehand drive (ball is not yet in her zone, but she's totally ready to start her forward swing), and serve (ball has reached its apex, she is ready to whip her racquet behind her back and spring up for the ball). This early preparation has a lot to do with being able to keep the ground stroke/service motion smooth, but also it has something to do with countering the tendency to hold back during pressure points. Same with your costal inhalation in preparation to speak.

Why a smooth, continuous diaphragm movement?

A good tennis stroke (or most any athletic motion) is, once begun, smooth and continuous. Trouble usually arises when there is any kind of stoppage of motion. Tennis coaches call this a 'hitch'. But it usually does not cause problems unless the player is under pressure. Why? Because tension (caused by the fear of losing) has a chance to get in and cause the muscles to tighten and sometimes freeze. This is called 'choking'.

Same thing with the diaphragm. If you allow it to stop at some point during its motion, the fear will take over and cause it to contract when it needs to relax. Again, this will generally happen when the pressure is on.

Now, there are two problems: one is that, because the diaphragm comes down before it goes up, there will always be a certain amount of stopping between the inhale and exhale. Your job is to make this 'hitch' as short as possible. Again, the only time the diaphragm perceptively stops moving is during the pause when your breath is out.

The other problem comes later when you are feeling a strong fluency but are not quite 'there'. As you become more spontaneous and automatic, you will tend to get sloppy with your diaphragm motion. When you get sloppy, your costal diaphragm is no longer moving smoothly from up to down to up. Or you might even be speaking for the crural diaphragm. There are all kinds of little hitches and blitches that will soon become habitual. This is called normal speech. Unfortunately, it is destructive to you because your fear in certain situations is greater than for non-stammerers. These little hitches give the fear a chance to freeze your diaphragm. This is called 'blocking'.

There will come a time when you can be sloppy, but not until you haven't blocked for several months. And when you do have a block (or series of) after a long period of fluency, you need to realise that it is primarily because your diaphragm motion is no longer smooth. This means that you will need to get down and do some hard work to work out the hitches.

Perhaps a good thing to remember is 'a rolling stone gathers no moss'. A moving diaphragm gathers no blocks.

The urge to be a totally normal speaker with normal bumbles, and stumbles, poor formulation, and unnecessary words will become quite overwhelming. Perhaps at first it will be like trying to keep a baby from being born. There is probably nothing that you or I or anyone can do to prevent it. However, after you've had your fling with normal speech, you would do well to continue your journey towards eloquent speech. A full, smooth from up-to-down-to-up diaphragm motion produces eloquent speech just like a full, smooth tennis stroke produces a good shot. Why not keep your diaphragm operating smooth and full and be an excellent speaker rather than a sloppy, normal speaker?

Why timing?

When it's time to speak, it's time to speak. And when is this? It is immediately after the full inhale/rib expansion. Not after a short pause after the inhale/rib expansion. Not after little release of air. (Remember, your diaphragm must move smoothly and continuously once it begins to move). Anything else is holding back making you more vulnerable to blocking.

When I was learning to give my old Bedford camper van (his name is Farkwar) a tune-up, I was amazed at the difference a small turn of the distributor made in his performance. Timing. He started easier, had more power, got better gas mileage, and didn't explode while the family was on vacation a thousand miles from home. Just the fourth gear went out, but would operate if I kept pressure on the gear-shift lever.

Why am I boring you with this? Because if and when you have trouble (many blocks per day and starting to use tricks), it will sometimes be a timing problem. Let's consult with Farkwar for an explanation:

Farkwar's engine: Piston goes down and draws in a mixture of gas and air. Piston moves up compressing the fuel mixture. Distributor sends a high voltage current to the spark plug that ignites the mixture causing a small explosion. The piston is forced down. Exhaust is expelled on the up stroke.

Now, the distributor has to be timed so that the spark reaches the fuel mixture at the exact right moment, which is when the piston is at the exact top of the stroke and ready to go down. Too soon or too late results in power loss, poor gas mileage and will eventually damage Farkwar's engine.

Your speaking engine: diaphragm contracts, then relaxes. It first moves down towards the abdomen, then up into the thorax. A vacuum is first created in your thorax, then released. Air is first drawn in, then expelled out. You inhale, then you exhale. You inhale, then you speak. Your words are like the spark in Farkwar's cylinders. Too soon or too late results in loss of power, weak elocution, and eventual damage to your fluency – namely big fat blocks.

The danger zone for you is between the inhale and the exhale. That is where you are most likely to block because your diaphragm must stop its downward motion before it starts moving upwards.

It must stop contracting before it starts relaxing. Unfortunately, it is impossible to have a completely smooth continuous diaphragm motion. No matter how hard you try, there will always be a 'blip' (stop) between the inhale and exhale. However, you can make this blip extremely short. Assuming everything else is also working properly, the shorter this blip/stop is and the quicker you begin to speak after the inhale/rib expansion the less chance you have of blocking.

But to make the blip extremely short, you must observe and practise. Just make sure you are exhaling/speaking immediately after your inhale. Again, this is one good reason for your hands on your ribs. The quick punch as you begin to speak/exhale helps perfect your timing. And this is why God made tape recorders, video cameras, mirrors and friends.

Why project your voice through your chest?
This whole process is ultimately to get your speaking process down in your chest rather than your mouth and vocal cords. Having your attention only in your mouth or throat while you are speaking is like a tennis player thinking only of his wrist or hand or racquet face. It will not hold up under pressure.

For we who stammer, it's too much attention in the mouth and vocal cords that is causing the problems. That is because most of your tricks are happening in your mouth and vocal cords.

Leave everything above your shoulders and below your forehead alone. Your mouth and vocal cords already know exactly what to do to speak. If you have your attention anywhere during the speaking process, get it down in your chest where the real action is. Above your forehead is your frontal cortex. That is where you deal with the fear.

Why lower your voice tone?
A deep, rich voice is one of the best tools for keeping your speaking process down in your chest. It is also more eloquent and powerful regardless if you are male or female. And again, it has to do with changing your speaking personality.

One thing, however, is you have to differentiate between a deep tone produced from the glottis and a deep tone from the chest. You can indeed produce a somewhat raspy, deep voice from the glottis but unfortunately, you are also putting focus on that area that will result in your vocal cords clamping shut when the fear hits. To make sure the deepness is coming from the chest, you have to pay attention especially on any tension in the area of the larynx. A deep tone from the thorax will be more breathy at first but will richen with practice. It would also be wise to listen to yourself regularly on a tape recorder.

Why assertive (even aggressive) first sound?
There is a sport in Holland where one must jump fairly wide, not-so-clean canals. The jumper must run very fast, jump very hard, grabbing a long pole that is loosely sticking upright in the canal. The jumper must climb the pole as his momentum makes the pole fall towards the far bank. If there is enough momentum and if the jumper climbs fast enough, the falling pole will drop

the jumper on firm ground. If the jump and pole climbing was not hard and fast enough, the jumper ends up in the not-so-clean canal.

Why did I just tell you this story? Because the same thing must happen when you're facing a feared situation. You are trying to jump over the fear. If the canal jumper jumps slow and cautious (holding back), he will get a cold, dirty bath. If you begin to speak in a feared situation with a slow and cautious (holding back) attitude, you will tend to freeze in the fear and get a cold, dirty block. Another analogy is jumping through a wall of flame. Assuming you know it is only a wall and not a room of flame, how do you jump? Slow and cautious, or fast and hard? Fast and hard, of course, otherwise you'll get fried.

Stammering, on the psychological level, is the act of holding back and avoiding while trying to speak. What is the opposite of this? Assertiveness, of course, and, in practice to overcome severe holding back, you should hit the first sound aggressively. Now, I'm not advocating becoming aggressive in your interpersonal relationships – although we will work on assertiveness later. What I'm talking about is aggressiveness in the breathing mechanics of speaking.

Fast, full, assertiveness/aggressiveness will usually get you through that first barrier in feared situations. Once you are rolling, you will usually be fine. If not, it just means you need to practise more. And you do indeed need to practise it so that it is there when you need it. Do not expect it to work if you don't practise.

Remember: This fast, full, aggressive attack kind-of-speaking is not supposed to sound natural. You don't need to do it in normal conversations except to practise. It is to counteract your habit of avoiding and holding back.

Don't be afraid to take a big step. You can't cross a chasm
in two small jumps.
David Lloyd-George

Why articulate?

To articulate is to be very precise in the way we speak. This means to enunciate and pronounce the words and sounds properly. Besides just being part of speaking eloquently, it is to make sure you are not using tricks. Many who stammer develop many gimmicks and fillers to get words out. Sometimes they leave out sounds. Or substitute sounds. Or try to 'skate' over blocks by using a soft contact. The final result is reinforcement of the avoidance behaviour that perpetuates stammering, and is anything but eloquent.

> *Most of the evils in life arise*
> *from man's being unable to sit still in a room*
> BLAISE PASCAL (1623–62)

So. You got it? Here is the whole shebang of what we call 'the cycle of powerful speaking'

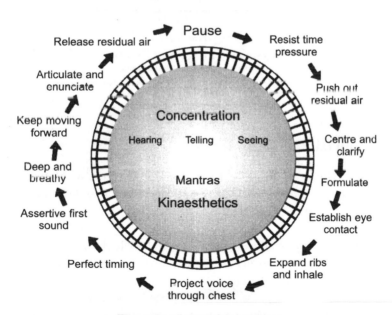

The cycle of powerful speaking
Playing to win rather than playing to lose

Levels of progress to eloquence

If you follow the directions, work hard and, later, be courageous, your progress from the swamp of out-of-control stammering (unbridled use of tricks and avoidance) to eloquence should be something like this:

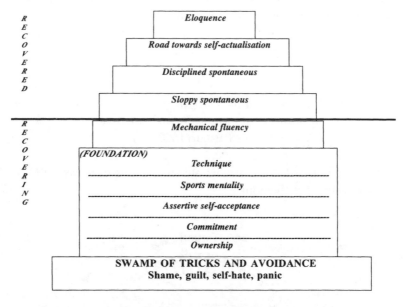

Levels of progress to eloquence

Explanations of the levels

Swamp: This is what brought you into the programme. Your stammer is out of control with the use of tricks and avoidance. Panic, guilt, shame, self-hate is high.

Foundation: You want a strong platform on which to develop your eloquence. As foundations are stronger when layered, this foundation comes in several levels:

- *Ownership:* Not only do you own your stammer (not someone else's problem), you own the responsibility to overcome it and become a strong speaker. No one else but you is going to do this. You own it and this is the first layer of your foundation.

- *Commitment:* Once you've taken ownership, you have to make a personal commitment to do something about it. It helps if you make this commitment to someone else as well.

- *Assertive self-Acceptance: You* have to assertively accept yourself as a recovering stammerer. This is an active process. You can not sit around self accepting, but, rather, go out of your way to show people you are a stammerer doing his/her best to become a strong, eloquent speaker. This means that deliberate dysfluency itself has to be taken to the boring stage. More will be said about this in Chapter Four.

- *Sports mentality:* Once you start seeing yourself as an athlete trying to get good at a sport – the sport of speaking – you stop seeing yourself as a victim needing 'treatment'. Athletes have to take responsibility for their own progress. So do you. Everything that it takes to become good at a sport (or musical instrument) is needed to become good at the sport of speaking.

- *Technique:* As in any skilled sport, proper technique needs to be learned and drilled before one can play a game.

Generally, if you're having more than your share of turbulence or chronically relapsing, one or more of your foundations layers are not solid.

- *Mechanical fluency:* Until the technique is automatic and all feared words and situations are overkilled, you should be sounding fairly mechanical using the 'Climbing Checklist' and not too many words per breath. This is a higher level of self-acceptance. You are being 'mechanical' because you are a stammerer and this is what you have to do to become a strong, eloquent speaker.

- *Sloppy spontaneous: You* might reach the orbit zone before you've grooved your technique. You will feel so free and fluent that it will be very difficult for you to be disciplined and stay in the mechanical stage. It's much like trying to keep a baby from being born. You will use virtually no technique and will probably be quite normally dysfluent. Congratulations! This means you have overkilled all your feared words and situations and are truly, albeit temporarily, free from stammering and on your way to eloquence. You will no doubt, however, take a fall from here back down to the swamp. Then you will have to rebuild your foundation, stay longer in the mechanical stage and hopefully go to the stage called:

- *Disciplined spontaneous:* this is where you don't really have to think about any technique for speaking, but the technique itself is habituated and is happening automatically. You have struck a nice balance between discipline and spontaneity. You are, by this point, quite articulate.

- *Road to self-Actualisation:* For most, self-actualisation is a life-time process. It is the process of overlapping your two circles so that what others see is what they get and you are realising your potential to do with this precious life exactly what you want to be doing and know exactly who you are in relation to the world and other people. The important thing is to be on the road to self-actualisation. This makes things you say very interesting to other people, and this leads to:

- *Eloquence: You* enjoy and feel what you are saying. Other people enjoy and feel what you are saying. And you do this with good voice tone and good articulation.

CHAPTER FOUR:

Dealing with the fear with concentration and fighting fire with fire. Breaking the cycle of panic

It's alright to have butterflies in your stomach.
Just get them to fly in formation.
DR ROB GILBERT

You now understand from the first two chapters at least our version of the psychology and physiology of stammering. You've learned the technique, drilled it into automatic habit, and understand why we do it. Now, it's ALMOST time to take it to the real world.

Not so fast. I said 'almost'. We like to think our technique is the best technique available, but even this will not hold up if you have too much fear that is bordering on (or diving into) panic. One of the things you need to do, like any athlete or musician, is concentrate. Concentration and panic don't go well together.

You've experienced intense fear and panic all your life when it came to speaking. This is most definitely not going to go away overnight. And perhaps, according to the experiments on the stickiness of fear-based learning (and stammering is most definitely fear-based learning), it may never go away completely, which is why no programme can promise you a cure. But there are things you can do to minimise it.

Remember the scenario with the double faulting tennis player at the start of the last chapter? The teaching pro first had to clean up the dysfunctional technique. If the tennis student is still double faulting even with good technique, a good coach will recognise the need to deal with the fear. The main tool a good tennis coach will use is concentration.

Concentration

In the last chapter we mentioned that development of concentration is one of the best tools for controlling fear, not to mention improving performance. Here are a few more things to think about and practise:

Replace the negative thoughts with positive: I recall my own tennis coach saying 'Don't make your service toss until the thoughts of double faulting are out of your head'. He made me wait, similar to what you are doing in your pause. Then he said, 'Repeat those things, silently to yourself, that you need to do to make a good serve'.

The idea was by repeating 'Bend your knees, arch your back, spring up at the ball, etc.' there would be no room for 'Better not double fault, what will my friends think if I double fault this game away too, etc.'

Turbocharging 'hearing yourself': that you do during your pause. Do a whole bunch of reading out loud, but before you say anything, make sure you've 'heard' it in your head before it comes out of your mouth. This includes 'hearing' the deep breathy tone. Practice this for at least a half hour, guiding yourself back to CONCENTRATION every time your mind wanders. This may get boring, like most concentration exercises, but keep at it with the idea that you are developing your powers of concentration for when you are out there in the trenches of the real speaking world.

Visual focal point
Another technique taught by my tennis coach was 'see the seams on the ball' or the pieces of fuzzy felt during the ball toss for a serve or as the ball was coming over the net for a volley or groundstroke. Another thing was to see the line between the dark and light side as the sun hit the ball. By concentrating on this, you control the fear and keep it from turning into panic, *and*, you get out of

the way of your body that knows exactly what to do to hit a good shot.

Same with speaking. Practise reading, or just talking to yourself, while *concentrating* on looking at the small reflection of light in your own eyes in the mirror. If you don't have a mirror handy, a dot, piece of lint, etc. will be enough to practise. The smaller, the better. Make sure you keep whatever it is in focus as you speak. When it gets out of focus, bring it back into focus. This takes concentration. The more you practise it, the easier, and more effective it will become.

Auditory focal point

Read aloud or find something to say where you can focus on the process rather than content. As you speak, focus your concentration on hearing your voice coming out of your chest (not your mouth or throat because we want to get attention away from there so that these muscles can do their job). When you're really in a tough speaking situation and the fear is high, feel it coming from your abdomen. Again, 'hear' the words in your head before you speak and 'hear' the words as they come from your chest or abdomen.

Visualisation

My trombone teacher said to visualise the sound going out the window into our neighbour's yard. My tennis coach said to imagine the ball leaving the sweet-spot of the strings and travelling, complete with spin and arch, to the exact spot I want it to go. Not only does that produce a better, more full sound on the trombone and greater accuracy and consistency on the tennis court, the intense concentration required also displaces the fear and keeps it well away from panic. Trick is to do it during a performance or match. But, of course, it takes practice beforehand. Lots of practice.

Looking at the pictures of the ribs and diaphragm in the second chapter, try to imagine the rib cage, as a unit, moving up and out and the diaphragm contracting downward while you inhale. Then the ribs moving, again as a unit, down and in and the diaphragm relaxing upwards as you exhale and/or speak. Takes a bit of practice and work, but you can do it.

Another simple thing to do, but one that requires the development of concentration, is to visualise the written words before and as you say them. ,

If you'd like a simple computerised image of ribs and diaphragm moving together, just drop an email to davetmcguire@msn.com and I'll show you where to find it on the net.

Mantra

When the pressure is on during a tough match, I have a little jingle (called in Zen circles a Mantra) to help keep away the double fault/easy shot blowing demons. Before serving, my mantra is: bend you knees, arch your back, see the ball, snap your wrist up and across the ball, go for the (backhand, forehand, body)'. When returning serve, I'll say to myself 'see the ball, turn shoulders, see the ball hit the strings, go down the line/crosscourt'.

Same with speaking. Once you get the image of the diaphragm and ribs moving together as you inhale and exhale, put it all to symbols (called words) with the following mantra:

> My ribs have just moved out and up, and the top of my
> diaphragm contracted downwards as my costal diaphragm
> contracted, which created a vacuum in my thorax, which
> sucked air into the alveoli of my lungs. But now, present
> tense, my ribs are moving down and in and my costal
> diaphragm is relaxing causing the top of the diaphragm to
> relax upwards, which releases the vacuum in the thorax
> causing air to pass over my vocal cords so I can speak.

Repeat this several time while imaging the ribs and diaphragm. Make sure the anatomy is synchronised with the words.

Tactile focal point

Feel your chest resonating as you speak. It helps to put your hand on your chest. Say something and concentrate on the vibration. Remember, give it enough time and concentrate.

Fighting fire with fire

Reducing the fear with Assertive Self-Acceptance: Deliberate Dysfluency and Disclosures. *"Showing and telling people who you are and what you are doing".*

If you can deal with the fear with concentration alone, GREAT! Most athletes do it this way. But we who stammer have some pretty traumatic experiences going around in our subconscious that make it difficult to accept ourselves for who and what we are. We have the habit of trying to hide who we are, and it is this hiding and deceiving that increases the fear and perpetuates the blocking.

Assertive Self-Acceptance

So we who stammer sometimes need to do something extra to control and extinguish this fear. This "something else" is to repeatedly do the very thing that frightens us the most. We need to actively and assertively show and tell people who we are and what we are doing which is: "a person who stammers trying to become a better speaker".

In many respects, this is much like fighting forest fires where stuff like grass, brush and trees is the fuel that feeds the fires. Fire fighters will create controlled fires called "backfires" to burn up the fuel ahead of the main fire. No fuel, no fire. No fear, no blocking.

Fear is indeed the fuel that feeds stammering. Where we run into trouble is when we try to pretend we are a totally normal speaker. This makes it very difficult to use any kind of good speaking technique, because, after all, a normal speaker doesn't have to use any technique. A normal speaker just talks. No costal breath, no pauses, no deep and breathy tone, no release of residual air. Just talk. It would be nice for us to be able to do this, but chances are you need, like any good athlete, to focus on technique. But we're afraid to do this because then we will not be seen as perfect.

How do we who stammer "light a backfire" to burn up the fear that is fueling the panic and blocking? It's already been said: SHOW AND TELL OTHER PEOPLE WHO YOU ARE AND WHAT YOU

ARE DOING! This is called "Assertive Self-Acceptance" and the two ways of doing it are Deliberate Dysfluency and Disclosing.

> *We are healed of a suffering only*
> *by experiencing it to the full.*
> MARCEL PROUST

Deliberate Dysfluency

And how do you show them? Simple. Just be very disciplined and mechanical in practicing the basic cycle of speaking, block release, hit and holds, just a few words per breath, etc, that you learned in the previous chapter whenever you speak even when you feel totally confident. Exaggerate everything. And to take it one step further, by making your hit and holds a bit longer and by doing two or three block releases, you are giving the listener the heads up that you are a person who stammers.

But remember: To truly make a backfire to burn up the fear, you have to exaggerate your discipline and exaggerate your hit & holds and block releases when you feel confident enough to be less exaggerated, and/or you don't need to use a block release or hit and hold.

If it looks like this is making your listener uncomfortable (or even if it isn't), then it's time for:

Disclosures

Just TELL THEM what you're doing and why. Get used to (and practice) saying something brief like:

"I'm recovering from stammering and have to concentrate on my breathing."
You might find yourself giving a lecture about the psychology and physiology of stammering which is good for you too ☺.

Talking about your stammer and what you are doing about it not only reduces your stress and fear, it is courteous to you listener. I can remember Dr. Sheehan telling the story about how a person who stammers talking with a fluent speaker is like having a conversation with a baby hippo under the table. Neither wants to acknowledge the hippo and things become very uncomfortable. Once someone, especially the person who stammers, says "hey, we got a baby hippo here under the table" ("I'm trying to overcome a stammer"), things lighten up. The listener, and thereby the stammering person, is put at ease thereby reducing the stress. The less the stress, the less the fear, and the easier it is to concentrate. Less stress = less fear = better concentration = better speech.

Remember, the big approach-avoidance conflict that we're all facing of "fear of stammering versus desire to be fluent", is more accurately the "fear of being seen as a stammerer, versus desire to be seen as a normal speaker".

A few more points on using Block Releases and Hit and Holds as Deliberate Dysfluency to show the listener you are someone dealing with a stammer.

- Deliberate Dysfluency is a mentality, not a technique. You are not doing this to get out a word or to be fluent. What needs to be foremost in your mind is: *"I'm gonna show this person that I am indeed a person doing something about a stammer."*
- Remember that you are being "proactive" rather than "reactive". You're attacking the fear of being seen as a stammerer rather than waiting for it to come to you. You are going after a difficult situation with the 'right' attitude, rather than waiting for it to come to you.
- When you use Hit and Hold and/or Block Release to show that you are a person who stammers, it's important that you do this on non-feared words. If used to counteract the distortion on feared words/sounds, it cannot be counted as 'pro-active' or deliberate. You're fighting the main fire, rather than lighting a backfire.
- When using the Hit and Hold, make sure it is long enough to let the other person know that you are indeed a person who stammers. Resist the temptation to pull out of it early. Exaggerate!
- Deliberate Dysfluency must be done with the full pause, costal breath, etc. Pay attention to your eye contact. The old habit of looking away will be very strong. Keep that tiny reflection in the other person's eye in focus.
- Your deliberate Hit and Hold might turn into a real block, which means the non-feared word became a feared word. You will have to overkill it to the boring stage like any other feared word. It also means that you have to do more Deliberate Dysfluency rather

than less. Resist the urge to think: "It's the Deliberate Dysfluency that caused me to block, so I'd better not try it anymore."

My personal experience with Deliberate Dysfluency
by Steve Sheasby

Four months into the programme, I still find Deliberate Dysfluency an incredibly useful tool. It seems crazy: most of my life I have tried to minimise my stammering (I should add not very successfully!) and now I am being told to stammer on purpose. Crazy, but it works.

It works in four ways for me at the present time. Firstly, it advertises to my listener that I am a recovering stammerer: a stammerer, but one that is not ashamed of his stammering. I can watch my listener's reactions (even mark them out of 10!); if they look away I stop immediately (as my primary coach Ray Worster advised) and wait until they re-establish eye contact. You see it puts me in the driving seat. Secondly, Deliberate Dysfluency is a very useful fear reduction tool. If I enter a situation and feel a little tense there is nothing like a few deliberate dysfluencies to get me on an even keel again. Thirdly, it is a great tool for self-acceptance (as a recovering stammerer). My fluency has greatly increased since being on the programme, and an obvious trap would be to think of myself now as a fluent speaker. I may understand this intellectually but I still need to actually do Deliberate Dysfluencies on a regular basis. And finally and fourthly, Deliberate Dysfluency is incredibly useful for practice: how else am I going to practice block releases, long hit-and-holds or short hit-and-holds in real life speaking situations? I need to practice these so that I am proficient in them for the times I need them for real. And I will need them; an odd word (and block) will occasionally apparently pop up from nowhere. So, there are four ways that Deliberate Dysfluency is working for me, but how do I actually do it?

There are four ways I use to add Deliberate Disfluency into my speech. Firstly, I use long hit-and-holds. Secondly, I use voluntary short hit-and-holds. Thirdly, I use exaggerated technique. This is an important one for me as it gives me a chance to practice all the points of the checklist in real life speaking situations, for example, I used to feel a terrible sense of hurry whenever I spoke, so what better way to counter this than with a long (and I mean sometimes a very long!) pause. The fourth and final way I include Deliberate Dysfluencies into my speech is with deliberate block releases. I always think of stammering as repetitive so deliberate block release is especially useful for me. Deliberate Dysfluency, at this early stage of my recovery, really needs SMART goals (Specific, Measurable, Achievable, Relevant, and Time-related). It's no good telling myself I'm going to try to put more deliberate dysfluency into my speech; I need to say, for example, that when I talk to my boss next time I will use two examples of Deliberate Dysfluency. Simple, but effective.

So, that's why I use Deliberate Dysfluency, and how I use it. Oh yes! And one more reason I use it: because it's FUN!

What to do with a feared word

Tools available for emergencies and overkill:

1. *Exaggerated deep tone:* You see the word from hell coming, but your fear is mild to moderate. Just hit it with a deep tone from the chest.

2. *Block release:* Handy little item for when you lose your train of thought, searching for a word, etc. and don't want to sit there with a half-contracted diaphragm. But it's also good for real blocks when they surprise you. You release the air, relax and push your diaphragm up into the relaxed position, pause to get it together, and give the word another try. Sometimes it is even okay to start at the beginning of the sentence again.

3. *Block release with deeper tone on the second try:* If the block is mild to moderately severe, you can release, make sure you pause, then hit it again with a deeper tone focusing on the sound coming out of the chest.

4. *Hit and Hold:* You're in the moderate to severe level of fear. Reread the section on Hit and Hold remembering that you are hitting the first sound because you are afraid of it and you are

prolonging the first sound because you are afraid of prolonging the first sound. You are doing what you are afraid of doing . . . good non-avoidance strategy.

5. *Hit and Hold with block release:* Fear has got more severe. You start holding back in the middle of the 'hold' and you feel it come to your mouth. Release it, pause, do another hit and hold making sure the second is also deep from the chest. You might have to do this a few times.

6. *Deliberate dysfluency on the words surrounding the feared word:* Of course, this is after you've tried the above. Start the sentence over and do some severe deliberate dysfluency before the word from hell then do a good hit and hold.

7. *Prolong past the block:* Looks as if it is firmly in the panic stage. You tried all the above. Your listener is patient and is willing to wait while you do battle. You probably have a terrible urge to use one of your old tricks or even word-substitute. Or you might even want to walk away. If you can keep it together, you might try the old Sheehan way, which is to prolong the sound past the block. This will take some guts. Be persistent.

Unless you have considerable experience or are exceptionally talented, these techniques will be difficult to use in a surprise situation. Just do the best you can then get down a.s.a.p., using these tools, to cancel and overkill these words to the boring stage.

Keep reminding yourself, as you read on, that the object of all this is to break that approach-avoidance conflict, break the cycle of panic, and to eat up the fuel of fear that is keeping you from concentrating on good speaking technique.

Overkill

You're getting close to taking this whole thing out to the real world. Although it can be counter-productive to view this whole thing as a war rather than a sport, there is one thing about war that applies to what you want to do, namely: dealing with a feared word or sound so that it is no longer feared. In this, it becomes more like a war than a sport, as very few sports take on the level of fear that you experience in the early stages of getting something as silly as a sound or word so it doesn't send shivers up your spine and sweat down your face.

So, just this once, let's look at it like a war. Basic to war is the concept of 'overkill'. Too much is better than not enough. That is what Sherman was doing when he made his infamous march to the sea during the American Civil War. That is what the politicians did *not* do during the Vietnam War.

Our 'enemy' is the fear. Or perhaps a better word is the panic. Fear of what? Panic from what? Well, fear of a sound or a series of symbols called letters that make up things called 'words'. Somewhere along the line, these silly symbols became super charged with fear, probably because you got major stuck and experienced a great deal of the all too familiar shame, guilt and self hate. Okay, we all know what this is but what to do about it? We'll talk about it more throughout this book: OVERKILL. Take the word or sound out to the street and to the phone and, starting with one word that gave you trouble in the easiest possible situation (quiet shop with a nice clerk or hotel for phone work) start overkilling the little bugger to what we call the BORING stage. But before you reach the luxury of 'boring', there are some other stages you go through:

Panic: Diaphragm, articulators and/or vocal cords are starting to freeze up. Fear is intense. Perhaps you're grabbing for those little tricks you use to get out a feared word or ways to avoid the word or ways to get out of the situation. Even in the easiest contacts with strangers, things are out of control every time.

Barely manageable fear: You've stayed disciplined and have been pounding the word and it's starting to give. Still, out of every ten contacts there is struggle in one or more of the three areas of speech production more than five times.

Exciting fear stage: You're still at it and things are looking up. Like taking the lead against a tough sports opponent who still has the capacity to come back and thrash you. Out of ten contacts, you are keeping it down in the chest with no struggle in the three areas more than five times.

Fun: Your 'opponent' is pretty much down and you have the game all but won, but will come back if you let up. Out of a hundred contacts it gives you trouble only once or twice.

Boring: You've won. Out of 100 contacts, everything stays solidly down in your chest. Now you have to be concerned with staying disciplined and not sloppy. Boring is good. It is a luxury. It means the absence of fear. When applied to feared words and situations, it is true freedom. Relish it.

Now go to the next word that gave you trouble during your turbulence. Chances are it surrendered after watching you beat up his big brother, but just in case, do about 10 to 20 contacts to make sure he doesn't want to come out and fight.

Honesty and the four fears

We sometimes say to new students just finishing their first course: 'you have been cursed with fluency'. Usually, their speech is very strong and sky high after making 100 contacts and public speaking on the third day of the course. But we have to caution them constantly that there is some situation out there waiting to surprise them. Perhaps the sight of an important person at a party coming for an introduction. Or making a call and someone unexpected picks up the line. Any such surprise stimulus can unlock the great flood of fear still stored in the unconscious plus some new ones:

- *The old fear of stammering. Such chronic fear will not go away overnight. But it will go away after you have proven you can deal with it, and it does not mean a return to uncontrolled stammering.*
- *Fear of losing fluency. If one has been fluent for a long time, this is probably the greatest fear of all.*
- *Fear of being perceived as a liar or foolish. Especially if you have told others that you are 'cured'.*
- *Fear of a repeat (and accompanying great disappointment) of relapse. This applies to those who have achieved and lost fluency in another program. The old 'here we go again' syndrome.*

Just be aware that your taste of freedom from stammering will increase the fear of losing it. Of these four fears, the most correctable is the one about having blown it by letting those around you think you are 'cured'. You'll have to go five years symptom-free before you can even think about 'cure'. In the meantime, enjoy your 'improving' eloquence, and let everyone know that you're still a 'work in progress'.

Other things to reduce the stress and fear

Realise that this costal breathing that you have committed to do at least twice per minute during your non-eating waking hours will relieve much of the stress related to the fear of stammering. So keep it up and even increase it.

There are many books on stress reduction. Just go to the book store or library and find one you like and follow its directions.

Taking it to the real world

You know what to do and hopefully you have a reasonable idea of why you do it. And you've drilled it enough that the whole thing is comfortable. And you have a reasonably good handle on how to deal with the fear, which, just like the physical stuff, needs to be practised and drilled.

Most of the time you were by yourself with a tape recorder and mirror, or maybe with a very trusted friend. It should be pretty comfortable. Now do two things:

- Write down a hierarchy of feared speaking situations, with the least feared (for example, talking to your cat), at the bottom, and the most feared (job interviews, cold call sales?) at the top. Be very specific.
- Start working your way up this list. But not too fast. It will not do you any good to destroy your confidence at this point. Just a baby step at a time. A good place to start is to call up trusted family and friends and tell them exactly what you're doing and openly and diligently practise your technique with them. Then go to calling hotels, say your name, and ask for a price of a single room. Or stores during the day, say your name and ask what time they open in the morning. In the evenings, best to call restaurants to ask simple, quick questions like opening and closing time, etc.

Again. Drill. Drill. Drill. No serious athlete goes into competition with a new technique that is half-baked.

Get some support

If you've done everything in this chapter to get a handle on the fear and panic, but things are still falling apart, remember what we said in Chapter One about being alone. You probably need the support of other people. Try to recruit friends and family, but remember that you have to be careful not to burn them out. You can also try to contact a stammering support organisation, and join one of their support groups. But be aware that not all stammering association support groups are into putting forth the effort that this programme requires for significant improvement.

CHAPTER FIVE

Centring and clarifying

Minimising the confusion that turns fear into panic. Self-actualising. Reaching your potential.

He who knows others is wise.
He who knows himself is enlightened.
ANON

What is verbal communication? Okay, you're using spoken words to convey something to a listener. But what are you conveying? Unless you can come up with something better, what you convey are feelings (emotions) and thoughts. These are the two main categories and both of these have to be clarified before you speak. And these two things are done either well in advance of speaking and t or during the speaking process itself during the pause. You know . . . that thing on the checklist that comes after resist time pressure and push out residual air.

Eloquence and self-actualisation

The goal of this programme, as already stated, is eloquence. Reaching a goal usually requires objectives. The spiritual objective, therefore, to the programme goal is self-actualisation. This is usually a lifelong process. The important thing is to be on the road to really knowing yourself, making yourself the most positive person you can be, and realising your potential. Such a person seriously engaged in this process is full of interesting things to say. Being interested in what you are saying is part of being eloquent. Perhaps more important is the self-awareness – and becoming the best person you can be is important to help you hold on to your fluency.

Now centring, clarifying and self-actualisation has to do with getting in touch with yourself – your real self – and presenting that real self to other people. Let me try to illustrate it with something from a fellow named John Harrison who I'll tell you more about later:

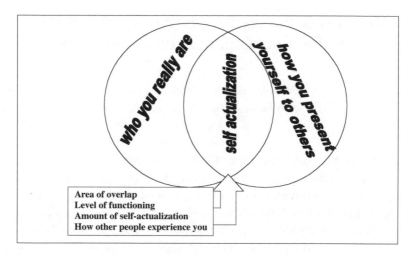

Self-actualisation (a)

The bigger the area of overlap, the greater the self-actualisation, the higher the level of functioning, the lower the stress, etc. The reverse is true for a smaller area of overlap.

'What you see is what you get'. Stress probably generally low. If such a person stammers, it is probably very mild. If circles continue to overlap more, stammering, even without the use of a technique, could very well disappear as it did with John Harrison. But, rest assured, it takes much work to get to this stage.

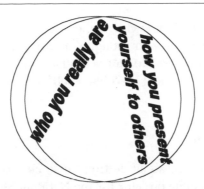

This person is "together", perhaps not perfect, but pretty much in tune with him/herself, portrays genuineness, promotes trust and honesty, commands respect, likes him/herself, etc You generally buy what's being sold. Pretty far down the road to self-actualization.

Self-actualisation (b)

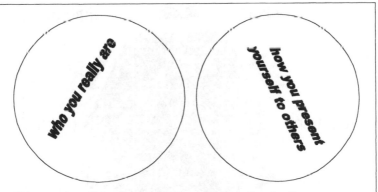

This person is totally out of touch with himself. No area of overlap. Keeps trying to sell the phoney self, but is oblivious to the fact that nobody's buying. Belongs in a "home". Stress might, in fact, be low.

Self-actualisation (c)

Man is the only creature
Who refuses to be what he is
ALBERT CAMUS

At first this is simply knowing, experiencing and accepting your feelings and clarifying your thoughts before you turn all this into words. This is the road to self-actualisation. One psychologist, Roberto Assegioli called it the 'higher self'. It is one of the by-products of this journey.

The Hexagon

So how does one go about getting those circles together? John Harrison, programme director for the National Stuttering Project, figured out that when all the components of oneself are functioning more in the positive than negative, fluency improves. He identified these components as intentions, behaviours, emotions, physical state, perceptions and beliefs. He then grouped them into what he calls the 'hexagon' with all components connected by lines thus:

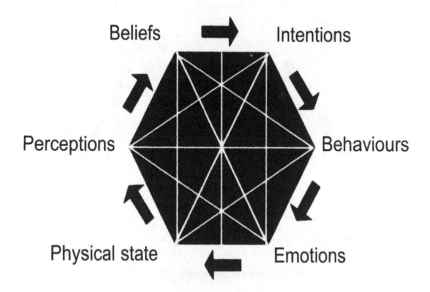

Your psychological and social system
(Harrison's Hexagon)

We, as living organisms are a system comprised by subsystems. There is a whole school of thought around systems as they apply to living organisms including human sociology and psychology. It's called systems theory. Now, I won't get into stuff like entropy, synthesis, steady state, homeostasis, etc. – or maybe I will. For now, Harrison's Hexagon is enough to get you going on systems.

If you look at the above model, you see the basic elements that make up your psychological and social being. And you notice that there are lines connecting one element to the others. So you get your first law of systems that says:

You don't go messin' with one part of the system without you messin' with the whole system!

Notice there are arrows pointing clockwise. This is to show the process of changing your hexagon (from negative to positive or visa-versa) starts with intentions, then goes to behaviours, and so forth. I'll explain more about this in a minute.

Law no 2 of the hexagon says: '**If you go messin' with one part of the system, you affect the other parts of the system, and, positively or negatively, affect the functioning of the whole system.**'

So part of centring, clarifying, getting those circles overlapping and moving towards self-actualisation – and probably the first step – is knowing your hexagon so you can see how everything fits together so that you can observe these components rather than 'be' the component. In other words, observing your fear rather than being your fear. So taking them in the usual order of change, let's look at each one:

Intentions

Intentions are intentions. It is what you tell yourself and others what you are going to do . . . and mean it. And a lot of times, it has nothing to do with words. It has to do with what you are really going to do. I mean REALLY do. What is important to remember is your intentions have to do with approach-avoidance conflicts. Remember, too, that an approach-avoidance conflict in one area of your life will lead to the fear of stammering approach-avoidance conflict. Get your intentions clear . . . make a decision and try to stick with it.

Behaviour

Well, maybe you have every intention in the world to do something. Or maybe you were just paying someone lip service. Whatever, your behaviour will say a lot about how sincere your professed intentions are. Ideally, your behaviour should always follow your intentions without a whole lot of procrastination. If this isn't happening you have an honour problem. You're not keeping your word to yourself and to others (see 'four traits of losing').

Emotions

We've all got them. And sometimes we need to convey them to someone else. Or sometimes we just need to know for ourselves what it is we are feeling. There are all kinds of emotions, good and bad. I'd like to talk about the good ones, but they aren't usually what gets us into trouble. Most of us have experienced a great increase in our fluency during the flush of love or excitement over something good that has or will happen to us. So let's talk about the not-so-gooduns like:

Anger: Pretty straight forward. Most of us know when we're mad. And expressing clear, righteous anger is one of the few times some of us who stammer have been totally fluent.

One problem with this is when we're not sure what it is that got us angry. Then we're confused and it's here that us who stammer get in trouble with our speech because of the old: fear + confusion = panic.

Another problem with anger is that, with some of us who have been brutalised because of our stammer, anger can quickly turn into rage. Rage is when you lose control and do and say destructive things that perhaps you regret later. Perhaps you are totally fluent when you are doing this damage, but the repercussions of destroyed relationships will later come back to cause you stress. And this stress will affect your speech.

Frustration: Something you feel when things don't work out the way you want. The important thing here is to be aware of it, do some relaxation things to control it, and don't let it turn into anger. Confusion has a lot to do with frustration.

Fear: for us who stammer, this is the biggie. The tendency has been for us to deny that fear and even run away from whatever is making us afraid. And sometimes, especially if you avoid it, that fear can turn into panic and terror. The idea is to admit you're afraid, feel where it is coming from (the general area of the diaphragm), and be courageous in facing it. In the words of Susan Jeffers 'feel the fear and do it anyway'. Then of course the old fear of fear + confusion = panic kicks in.

Part of this is accepting, too, that you have to deal with the fear.

Physical state:

This has to do with your body. You know . . . that collection of biological cells and chemical interactions that falls down when you step on a banana peel or your kid's roller skate. You know that usually 'more-trouble-than-it's-worth' thing that we never seem to keep proper care of. It's more significant than you think in terms of influencing the rest of your hexagon. For our purposes, we think of it as providing the energy to do things whether it be washing the dishes, going to work or cleaning up a feared word.

Think of how it was when you last felt sick or hung over or jet lagged, or very tired. Chances are, your self-perception and belief in yourself weren't so good. And of course that didn't do your emotions, behaviours and intentions any good either. Then, naturally, you ran into major difficulties with your speech.

Perceptions

This is to do with how you see and interpret things in the here and now. You can, for example, perceive someone suffering from the 'flu who walks by you without saying hello as having contempt for you, or as someone simply having a hard time for whatever reason. Whether you see the acquaintance as someone contemptuous towards you or suffering from some physical or emotional upset will depend many times on the rest of your hexagon.

Beliefs

You can say, perhaps, that beliefs are simply perceptions that have been proven true over time. You believe that these perceptions will always be true. Your beliefs are the most powerful long-term influence on your hexagon and must be continually challenged. Your beliefs will be the last thing to change you as you deal with the rest of your hexagon. And, perhaps, it's your beliefs that are the beginning of change . . . it's called 'hope'. Another thing about beliefs is that they can be passed on from generation to generation within a family. Negative beliefs (and perhaps some positive ones) always need to be challenged.

Another thing is how do you change your hexagon from negative to positive. Well, other than simply being aware of the hexagon and the process, you need to look at those arrows that start with intentions, then behaviour all the way around to 'beliefs'. Start with your intentions and make sure these intentions are backed up with your behaviour. Here's a little tennis story to illustrate this:

Tennis and the hexagon

If you start playing tennis, you will first have to drill the proper technique until it is automatic before you get into real competition. Once you start playing competitive matches, it will boil down to things like mental toughness, concentration under pressure, fighting spirit, persistence . . . you know . . . all those things that have to do with character. It also has to do with the hexagon. Here is an example:

I just played the first clay court team tournament of the season. I won my singles match against a much younger, higher-ranked player. Surprised the hell out of me since I woke up feeling terrible from something I ate the night before. So looking at my hexagon, I went into my match with my body (physical state) feeling terrible. And, boy, did that affect my:

- Emotions (depressed)
- Perceptions ('I've never been able to win when I feel like this')
- Beliefs ('I've never been able to win when I feel like this')
- Behaviour (initially, poor concentration, poor preparation, lazy footwork,
  resulting in many unforced errors).

Important for my overcoming all this were my 'intentions' when I made up my mind that I was going to just do my best and see what happens. I forced myself to replace the negative perceptions and beliefs with positive ones and kept repeating all those things that I need to do to play well – 'see the ball', 'turn the shoulders', 'move the feet', 'run for everything', 'fight for every point', 'close

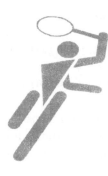

in after the drop shot' etc. until it became a mantra not allowing negative thoughts to enter.

Now, also important is the fact that I had practised hard all week with the intention that I was going to do my best to play well. I doubt that without this hard work put in to prepare myself that the positive thinking by itself could have overcome the effects of a body that felt miserable.

So the formula would go something like:

Positive, clear intentions + good preparation (practise and hard work) + persistence = more positive hexagon + improved performance + a good match + possible victory.

It is amazing how everything changed in the match. I soon perceived and believed that I could win, I was no longer feeling depressed and my body felt great.

Looking at my opponent, he was pretty cocky at first since I was the oldest by far on the team (they call me 'the old man') and looked pretty tired, plus I'm still a bit fat. His perceptions were 'there's no way I can lose to this guy', his beliefs were 'I've always beaten old guys like this especially if they're a bit fat'; his emotions: cocky over his upcoming victory; intentions were to beat me, but to make it look easy as someone on his level is not suppose to have too much trouble with a tired, fat old man. And his behaviour was to not concentrate as much as he should, and to over-hit the ball in an attempt to blow me away.

Towards the end of the second set (I had come from behind to win the first) you could almost see his hexagon changing. Because he couldn't blow me away, his intentions were in conflict (paralysis), he started making stupid mistakes, started thinking more about what his team-mates would think of him losing to the old man or even having the old man take him to three sets . . . stopped believing in himself. Played increasingly bad. Lost.

So what's the darn point. Simple. The hexagon, as stated, affects most all performance especially if you are under pressure. When you are speaking, you are, in a sense, performing – many times under pressure. Here are some points to remember:

- If your hexagon is more positive than negative, your performance will be better.
- If your hexagon is more negative than positive, your performance will be not as good.
- If your hexagon is in the positive, figure out what you did to get it there and what to do to hold on to it. Chances are things are going fine, but watch out for these things that we'll talk about more later:

arrogance – 'I am so unbelievably good, (not to mention good looking and cool) I can't lose. Furthermore my opponent is a real turkey. I, on the other hand, am cool. Thems who are cool always wins over thems who are turkeys.'

complacency – 'I got a great lead, just a few more points and I got him. There's no way I can lose. Therefore I don't have to really concentrate or fight for every point.'

- If your hexagon is in the negative, look at your intentions first, make the commitment, then make sure your behaviour follows the commitment. The rest of your hexagon will follow. You may not be perfect and you may block, but you will have given yourself the best possible chance to speak (perform) well. In getting your hexagon from negative to positive, pay attention to:

denial – 'I really don't have to make a major change in my game to win, I'll win because magic is on my side.'

intellectualisation – 'Wanting to win a tennis match/speak well is for those who aren't secure in themselves, therefore I don't really have to try my best.'

So make sure your intentions are clear and positive (even if you don't feel like it) if you want to keep your hexagon positive or quickly change it to the positive. Then make sure your behaviour supports your intentions. Keep your promises to yourself and others. Doing what you say you will do is all about honour.

Assertiveness

You, if your stammering was out of control, have probably been a juicy target for manipulators. The main weapon of a manipulator is confusion. He or she will count on you: (1) being unsure you're being manipulated; (2) not knowing how to deal with the manipulation. You then get caught in one or more approach-avoidance conflicts. And then your stuttering goes out of control.

> *He that always gives way to others*
> *will end in having no principles of his own.*
> AESOP

So why learn assertiveness? Six reasons:
(1) Stammering is the act of holding back when you speak. Assertiveness is the opposite of holding back. By moving forward (being assertive) in other areas of your life will help you to stop holding back while speaking.
(2) Becoming more assertive will help you from becoming confused when you run up against a manipulator (confusion + fear = panic).
(3) Knowing how to be assertive will help you to stop your manipulating of others . . . and will keep you out of the desire to be seen as honourable, fear of being seen as dishonourable approach avoidance conflict. It's all part of 'Centring and clarifying'.
(4) To be assertive with what you need to do to get good at speaking.
(5) To help you be assertive with yourself, and stop manipulating yourself out of working hard and being brave.
(6) Being assertive is one of the best ways to protect your emotions which, in turn, strengthens your whole hexagon.
I'm not going to try to teach you assertiveness here. Manuel Smith wrote an excellent book called *When I say no, I feel guilty* that you can get in almost any bookstore. He gives you a good description of what he calls your 'assertive rights' and teaches 'assertive skills' which are the tools to protect your rights and your boundaries.

But we do have a few things related to assertiveness and getting good at speaking thanks to Maree Sweeney, former Regional Director of the Irish programme. Here they are:

Assertive rights of recovery

1. *I have the right to use my full technique*
A manipulator will make you think that the full technique is not normal way of speaking. And that 'manipulator' may very well be you.

2. *I have the right to pause and take my time*
Other people, and/or you, may try to get you to think that you must hurry and it is wrong to keep them waiting.

3. *I have the right to take whatever time it takes for me to recover*
Other people, and/or yourself, may try to convince you that you have a time limit to reach a certain level of proficiency at this sport of speaking.

4. *I have the right to be selfish and to concentrate in working on my speech*
You, or someone else, might try to get you to believe that other things are more important than working on getting good at speaking.

5. *I have the right to make contacts as long as I show consideration for my listener*
You, or someone else, might try to convince you that going up to strangers and calling strangers to work on your speech is wrong.

6. *I have the right to overcome my stammer and to become a strong speaker, which means making mistakes but learning from these*
You, or someone else, might try to get you to believe that being a stammerer is a bad thing. Or someone, including maybe yourself, may try to convince you that it is wrong to want to overcome stammering.

7. *I have the right to go for fluency or non-fluency using deliberate dysfluency*
Someone trying to manipulate you or you manipulating yourself will try to get you to believe that going for fluency is wrong, or that deliberate dysfluency is wrong.

8. *I have the right not to care about other people's opinion and their judgment about overcoming stammering*
You and/or someone else will try to convince you that not caring about other people's opinion about what you are doing to improve your speech is wrong.

Fallacies of logic: the manipulator's key weapons to create confusion

Forewarned is forearmed. My mother sent me something years ago while I was in college called 'fallacies of logic'. It was, basically, a list of things a manipulator will do to twist things to manipulate others into thinking the manipulator is right and the other persons (including you) are wrong. Once this is done, they can get what they want, which is (usually) getting you to do what you don't want to do.

One of the effects upon your good self is that skilful use of fallacies of logic will confuse you. And confusion will lead to holding back – and holding back will lead to blocking as the all too familiar 'fear plus confusion = panic' sets in. Then of course, unless you are especially tough and assertive, the manipulator will get you to do what they want.

So the importance of reading further and learning this stuff is to be able to recognise when you are being jerked around by a manipulator. You might or might not want to confront the turkey, but at least you'll know what is going on and can stay centred and clarified.

1. *Unqualified generalisation:* No proof (facts)

2. *Hasty generalisation:* Too few instances to support conclusion

3. *Cause has no connection with effect*

4. *Contradictory premises* (If there's an irresistible force, there can be no immovable object). When the premises of an argument contradict each other, there can be no argument

5. *Substitution of sympathy appeal in place of pertinent statements*

6. *False analogy:* Different situations

7. *Hypothesis contrary to fact:* Conclusions are not supportable by hypothesis

8. *Poisoning the well:* Done by first speaker verbally attacking opponent

To understand how these work, it is important to read through these dialogues contributed by Australian graduates Bill Fabian and Andrew Cherinth.

Fallacies of logic . . . Eight examples (Author, Bill Fabian)
Bill tells his drinking buddy Dave, a confirmed bachelor, that he's going to marry Kerrie.
Bill: 'I've finally made a decision. I'm going to marry Kerrie.'
Dave: 'Are you mad ? Marriage is every man's downfall.'

1. *Unqualified generalisation: no proof, no facts.* Dave has fixed ideas about marriage that he thinks apply to everyone.
Bill: 'What makes you say that?'
Dave: 'Some of the blokes in the pub who were married tell me things.'

2. *Hasty generalisation: too few instances to support conclusion.* Dave only refers to the experiences of a few of his friends that he thinks will support his argument.
Bill: 'How do you mean?'
Dave: 'You know those alcoholics who are the first into the pub and the last out. All of them were married once and are now either divorced or separated. See where an unhappy marriage can lead you.'

3. *Cause has no connection with effect.* Dave implies that marriage leads to alcoholism, when the truth is that alcoholism is a physical addiction to a substance that often leads to divorce.
Bill: 'So you reckon their wives drove them to drink, eh?'
Dave: 'But worse still, my mates who are still married don't come down to the pub at all any more. They're really under the thumb.'

4. *Contradictory premises. When the premises of an argument contradict each other, there can be no argument.*

Dave assumes that because his mates aren't coming down to the pub that they are being controlled. The actual fact is that they probably have better things to do than go down to the pub.

Bill: 'I've got other things in life besides drinking at the pub, you know Dave.' Dave: 'Well what about me? It won't be the same if my best friend gets married. I'll only have those damned alcoholics to drink with.'

5. *Substitution of sympathy appeal in place of pertinent statements.* Dave appeals to Dave's sense of loyalty to an old friend.

Bill: 'I'm sure I'll find time to meet up with you for a drink now and then.'

Dave: 'Look Bill. Remember that time you bought that pet dog for a companion. He chewed up your furniture and crapped on your carpet. He made your life so miserable that you couldn't stand him. It'll be the same thing having a wife around, doing things you don't like.'

6. *False analogy: Different situations.* Dave makes an illogical comparison between two types of live-in companions.

Bill: 'I think she's house-trained Dave.'

Dave: 'I can ask out any woman I want and you'll be going home to the same one every night. You must be some kind of masochist.'

7. *Hypothesis contrary to fact: conclusions are not supportable by hypothesis.* Dave assumes his view of monogamy is shared by Bill and wrongly dismisses Bill's point of view as being one of self-hate.

Bill: 'That's true Dave. You do ask a lot of women out, but none of them ever says "Yes".'

Dave: 'Bill, I say this as a friend. I've known you for years. You always make wrong decisions. Marrying Kerrie will just confirm that you really are a pathetic loser.'

8. *Poisoning the well: Done by first speaker verbally attacking opponent.* Dave tries to give Bill doubts by ridiculing Bill's track record and attacking his credibility in making decisions.

Fallacies of logic: Eight examples from Andrew Cherinth

Now, a logical fallacy is an argument that has some defect in its reasoning.

1. '*Since unemployment in Australia is currently about 7 per cent, it must be about 7 per cent in the rest of the world as well.*' Every country is different, with the current states of their economy, the policies implemented by their governments and central banks and with their prospects for the future.

'Since we require oxygen to survive, all life-forms anywhere in the universe require oxygen.'

(One commonly held theory that I don't agree with).

2. *A hasty/sweeping generalisation makes a generalisation from a sample that is too small to support the conclusion.* 'Jim put his baby to sleep on her side, and she suffered SIDS. Sleeping babies on their sides causes SIDS.' 'The growing number of incidents of teenage suicides is an indication of the decline of teenage job prospects.' Of course small samples tend to be unrepresentative, and it's usually obvious when your sample space isn't large enough to make a fair appraisal. Statistics (mean, median, standard deviation, 5-year average, rate of change etc).

Although it seems improbable that people could successfully use arguments such as these, I've seen it happen, usually by extremely quick and confident speakers, who say it and draw a conclusion almost before you have time to think. Then they are drawing a conclusion and moving on to the next point, before you have a chance to jump in with 'Hey! Wait a minute . . .'!

3. *These arguments misidentify the cause of an issue.*
(i) Post-hoc – assert that an earlier event caused a later event simply because it happened earlier:
'I beat my drums during the solar eclipse and the gods spit the sun back . . . it works every time!'
(ii) You just identify one of many causes, and ignore the rest (over-simplification):
'I can't do well in school because I have a bad teacher.' How about the fact that you don't listen in class, don't do homework and don't study for exams?

4. *Sometimes an apparently good argument may be put forward, but may be inherently false when examined properly. For example consider the argument:*

'Temperatures have been rising through the more than 100 years we have been taking measurements. It's human activity, dumping carbon into the atmosphere, that's causing global warming.'

By itself, this seems reasonable enough. However when you consider that most of the temperature rise was before 1940 and that most of the carbon dumping has been post-1940, it contradicts the point the argument is trying to make. Or the statement, 'God, in his infinite compassion, sends sinners to hell for an eternity of damnation.'

Infinite compassion, yet infinite damnation! Where's the infinite compassion/forgiveness now?? Sending people to an eternity of torture hardly seems compassionate to me. Hence the contradiction, and the argument is meaningless.

5. *I would extend sympathy to 'appeal to emotion' with a number of subcategories.*
(i) Appeal to force: Use force or the threat of it to gain agreement on the part of the listener:

'If you want to keep working here, you'd better reconsider your criticisms of company policy.'

Of course coerced agreement is meaningless.
(ii) Appeal to pity – someone's distressed state/disadvantage/unfortunate occurrence used in an effort to persuade:

'I hope you agree that Michael Kasprowicz is the greatest fast bowler ever, we've spent all our money putting our museum together.'

i.e. Focus on the content of the argument, not his situation.
(iii) Appeal to popularity – The 'Bandwagon' fallacy, something surely everyone has been guilty of at one stage or another, the 'mob' mentality, i.e. assert that the more people or institutions that support your proposition, the more likely it is to be correct. Classic example, Columbus being attacked: 'The Earth must be flat. Millions of people know that it is. Are you trying to tell them that they are all mistaken fools?'

– Just because lots of people believe it, doesn't mean it's true. Have the guts to stand up for what you believe in. The worst that can happen is you'll be wrong. Nothing bad in that.

6. *False analogy – involves comparing two things known to be alike in one or more features and suggest that they are alike in other features as well.*

'What do you mean smoking is bad? Too much of anything is harmful. Too much apple-sauce is harmful.'

'We have pure food and drug laws; why can't we have laws to keep movie-makers from giving us filth?'

Alike in some ways does not necessarily lead to alike in all. You need to compare two things or ideas that have major relevant parallels in the aspects under consideration. Sometimes quick speakers can use this successfully as well.

7. *The argument from ignorance – since something has not been proven to be false, it can be assumed to be true.*
'Since you cannot prove that ghosts do not exist, they must exist.'

You can't base conclusions on what is unknown, a proposition may be true, false or pending. After you make one assumption that can lead to a whole new line of argument leading to a new conclusion, but it may all be based on a false assumption. So if someone tries to work off an unproven statement, pull the rug from under their feet.

It's interesting that this happened to Andrew Wiles, with his proof of Fermat's last Theorem. He actually had it solved back in *1996*, but had made an assumption regarding elliptical curves. Since the proof is hundreds of pages long, it took a while for someone to realise that the proof wasn't necessarily true. He then had to wait two years for a leading professor to prove that his assumption (regarding a theorem of elliptical curves) was true, and only then was his proof officially recognised. The point is that if it turned out to be false, he would have wasted years of work, not to mention showing everyone his approach to the proof, which he had guarded with unbelievable fervour (he worked for years in his attic, and no one was ever allowed in there, he was paranoid someone would beat him to the proof!)

8. *Attacking your opponent personally is done to change the subject, usually done to go to a more 'winnable' argument; hence it would be used when the manipulator falls on the back foot.* I.e. if you can't argue against the merits of another person's position, go after his character or weakness. It is attempted intimidation. What I found personally was that people after they felt threatened by my arguments began to mock me about my stammer, because prior to

the McGuire Programme that almost always had a huge effect on me. Unfortunately this often 'got to me', and the other person squirmed away. Or else something like 'Why should I care what you say? It's obvious that atheists like you have no moral values.' That didn't have any effect, but I've now learnt to just say: 'Let's get back to the topic at hand'. So if this happens, it's good, because you have the upper hand!

Related to this is when people refer to a third person/authority figure to say that their belief must be true because these experts or eminent scientists/ high-ranking members of the church hold the same belief. 'Patriarch John is the head of the Russian Orthodox Church, and he believes in original sin.' This was one used against me. My response, maybe a bit rude, was 'who cares?' Make up your own mind. I am especially sceptical when people cite an expert commenting about a topic outside of his area of expertise. This is another (attempted) change of subject, moving away from their stating their reasons for what they 'believe'.

What to do before a tough situation? Centring and clarifying flow chart

Even the strongest of our graduates will be thrown by certain situations that have a nasty combination of negative emotion and confusion. To unconfuse yourself, memorize the following flow chart and make a copy of it to keep handy.

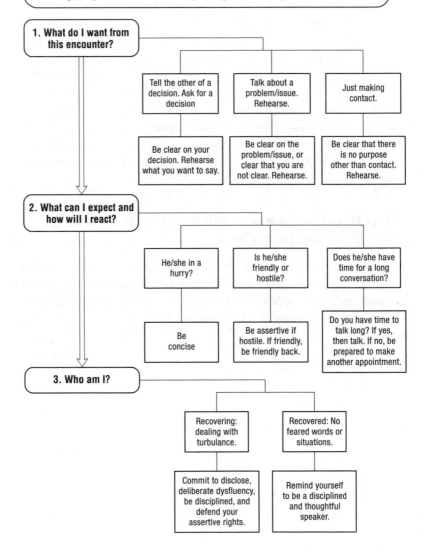

TOUGH SITUATION CENTRING AND CLARIFYING

Okay. Tough phone call or face-to-face encounter coming up? Do you just grab the phone/walk in and start babbling? Not a good idea. You may not block, but you might very well stick your foot in your mouth and come off like some kind of fool. Of course you've warmed up by being disciplined all day, made some extra contacts, etc., but now it's right before the encounter. Time to sit back for 3 to 5 minutes, breathe, close your eyes and center and clarify. Walk yourself through the following:

1. What do I want from this encounter?

| Tell the other of a decision. Ask for a decision | Talk about a problem/issue. Rehearse. | Just making contact. |

| Be clear on your decision. Rehearse what you want to say. | Be clear on the problem/issue, or clear that you are not clear. Rehearse. | Be clear that there is no purpose other than contact. Rehearse. |

2. What can I expect and how will I react?

| He/she in a hurry? | Is he/she friendly or hostile? | Does he/she have time for a long conversation? |

| Be concise | Be assertive if hostile. If friendly, be friendly back. | Do you have time to talk long? If yes, then talk. If no, be prepared to make another appointment. |

3. Who am I?

| Recovering: dealing with turbulence. | Recovered: No feared words or situations. |

| Commit to disclose, deliberate dysfluency, be disciplined, and defend your assertive rights. | Remind yourself to be a disciplined and thoughtful speaker. |

The more approach-avoidance conflicts, the more severe the stammer

PART TWO:

How to keep it

To be successful in this programme you must do your best to work hard, be courageous and persevere in following these directions:

Direction no. 1: Breathe from the costal diaphragm all day long except when you're eating. This should be no less than one costal breath per five normal breaths.

Direction no. 2: Speak with at least the basic method (pause, full costal breath, deep through the chest) whenever you speak.

Direction no. 3: Cancel poor technique.

Direction no. 4: Overkill your feared words to the boring stage.

Direction no. 5: Keep pushing out your Comfort Zone by challenging your feared situations.

> *Even if you're on the right track,*
> *you'll get run over if you just sit there.*
> WILL ROGERS

CHAPTER SIX:

Practice

Practice is the best of all instructors.
PUBLILIUS SYRUS

Tennis and speaking

As with golf, skiing, and learning almost any musical instrument, tennis is not one of those sports you can just go out, pick up a racquet and expect to play well. As in skiing where you have to train yourself to do unnatural things like putting all your weight on the downhill ski and leaning downhill (when your natural instincts are screaming to put your weight on both skis or the uphill ski and lean uphill), tennis requires you to do some things that aren't really natural and must be taught.

For example: the natural tendency is to hit the ball flat as you would a baseball. Or to swat the ball using your wrist and arm as you would in squash. Someone, generally, has to teach you that you must get your racquet under the ball to impart topspin and to lift the ball over the net and still have a degree of power. Someone also has to teach you to keep a firm wrist and turn your hips and shoulders so that you can torque energy that will produce controlled power.

Then we would also have to start talking about the why and what of grip changes between backhand, forehand, volley, and serve. Oh yes . . . ah . . . then we would have to teach you about bending your knees and moving your feet. But wait a minute, then we have to get into how to hit an approach shot when you see that short ball, not to mention the topspin lob, overhead smash, flat and spin serves, the slice backhand, down the line passing shot, sharp angled topspin winner, and, finally, the drop shot. But wait! Then what to do when your opponent hits you a drop shot? I think that's about it.

Then all these strokes have to be drilled until the techniques involved become automatic. All this comes under the heading of 'technique', which has to be mastered before you even start playing a competitive match. All this takes practise

The two habits

Just to remind you, there are two things in your new way of speaking must become automatic habits. The basic technique (with all its components) of speaking deeply through the chest with a full costal diaphragm must become a habit. Assertiveness non-avoidance including resisting time pressure and attacking feared situations must become a habit. For these to become habits, you must practise.

> *Bad habits are like a comfortable bed,*
> *easy to get into,*
> *but hard to get out of.*
> ANON

You must practise at least enough to have a steady improvement. If you are not improving, you must increase your practice time until you show steady improvement. Defeating stammering must become one of your life's top priorities. There are two things that must become automatic habits. The first is the physical technique of the basic cycle of speaking with all its components The second is the mental stuff including assertive self-acceptance, resisting time pressure, concentration under pressure, etc. For these to become habits, you must practice.

The horrible hundred

So what do you do in those two or more hours? After much trial and error, we found the most effective way to fill those two or more hours is by making at least 100 face-to-face or phone-to-phone contacts with strangers.

One hundred or more contacts a day will test your motivation. It is not easy. You will have to push yourself especially at the end to reach it. One hundred or more contacts a day does not leave room to sit around intellectualising and avoiding. You have do it fairly fast, otherwise you will stay up past your bedtime.

You gain strength, courage and confidence by every experience
In which you really stop to look fear in the face.
You are able to say to yourself,
'I lived through this horror. I can take the next thing that comes
along.'
You must do the thing you think you cannot do.
ELEANOR ROOSEVELT

For those of you who still think this is unreasonable and unfair, imagine yourself on a football team. The coach tells you to run laps after practice when you are already tired. You come to him saying, 'Sorry coach, I'm just too tired to run twenty laps. It's unfair and unreasonable for you to demand this of us. Ten is enough for me now.'

Any good coach would not even argue. Their response would be: 'Clean out your locker and do not come back.' Period.

Good news and bad news: The bad news is that you have to keep doing 100 situations a day until you reach the freedom of solid fluency where all words and situations are unfeared. The good news is that if you do 100 new contacts in addition to everything else, you will reach freedom quickly.

Why quantity?

It has been argued that it is better to have fewer but longer contacts. Not necessarily true. Generally, anyone – even a stranger – willing to give you more than a few minutes will have patient ears. Your fear level soon drops. This is fine for habituating the technique, but it is doing almost nothing for habituating your non-avoidance and assertiveness.

We are what we repeatedly do.

Excellence, then, is not an act,
but a habit.
ARISTOTLE

It has been initial contacts with strangers that have given you the most trouble in the past. You do not know if that new voice on the telephone or that new face in the street will be friendly or hostile. Understanding or teasing. Patient or irritable. You have thousands of examples of facing these situations with tricks and avoidance. You need thousands of examples of facing these unknowns with dignity and assertiveness.

Good news and bad news: First the bad news. Strangers on the phone and in the street have generally given you the most trouble in the past. You will, therefore, probably experience much fear at first. The good news is that, because you will never see these strangers again, these contacts will become quickly unfeared.

The phone and the street

So you've committed to going beyond stammering to articulate eloquence. You have declared total war in this fight for freedom. The best places to start habituating your new technique and assertive mentality is with strangers on the telephone or in the streets and shops. These situations are your 'war games' and practice matches.

These situations represent the lower part of your iceberg above the surface. There is no real consequence in dealing with strangers whom you will never see again. However, there is enough pressure involved to prepare you for the important tournaments.

Phone
If you live in a low population area, you might want to get Yellow Pages from surrounding areas. Warm up by asking for something using deliberate dysfluency on non-feared words. When you can do this fluently deep through the chest as well as with smooth deliberate dysfluency, start throwing in some feared words.

If the feared word is not something you can fit into the encounter, make up a fictitious name using that word. Perhaps it is the word 'direction'. Make up a name using that feared word. You can perhaps use the French pronunciation to make it seem more like a last name. 'This is Dan Direction. Can you tell me the price of a single room for tonight? Yes, it is an unusual name. Thank you.'

The best places to call early in the morning are hotels. Someone will always pick up the phone and not be angry at being bugged so early. Later on in the day, you can call shops. In the evening restaurants are good targets, but make sure you call back to cancel any reservations. In both shops and restaurants, it is best just to ask the opening or closing times. Again, the important thing is to get that feared word down in the chest with as many new voices as possible – this means many short contacts.

Get some newspapers. You will find the numbers of many businesses waiting for you to call. They are trying to sell things. After first saying your name, ask them about the punctured waterbed, the comic books, the chain saw, the bicycle. Ask its condition. Ask if they will take a lower price for them and say you will call back. Call them back. Say your name again then say you are not interested. Thank them for their time

If you run out of want-ads, restaurants and hotels in the evenings or holidays, you can call private numbers. Just be aware that you are bothering people in their own homes so, out of common courtesy, make it quick. Best to say your name and ask for the (feared word) pub, shop, office, etc. Your victim will quickly inform you that you have a wrong number. Just apologise, and go on to the next number.

Now, if you're especially stout-hearted, you can say something like: 'My name is (perhaps a feared work fictitious name). I've chosen your name out of the phone book at random because I'm trying to complete an assignment to help me recover from stammering. Could I have a minute of your time?' They will either tell you where to shove it, or give you the time. The originator of this exercise (Heather Lucy) reports many delightful conversations with people who become very interested in stammering and wanting to help.

Street

Find a good-sized town or city. Go to the busiest streets. Go into the shops and go up to people in the street. Warm up by asking for things while deliberately dysfluent on non-feared words.

Then start using your feared words. Ask for the (feared word) museum. The (feared word) pub. Try to avoid asking for an actual location – you do not have time to stand and listen to directions. And some sweet grandmother might lead you by the hand to a place you do not want to go.

For those who have reached a certain level of confidence the best thing to say is: 'Excuse me. I am a stammerer on a speech therapy course and my assignment is to tell a hundred people my name. I am (your name). Thank you for listening.' Of course, you should be using some deliberate dysfluency with this one.

Life is like playing a violin in public
and learning the instrument as one goes on.
SAMUEL BUTLER

The fifteen-minute sprint drill

Back in my high-school football days, the linemen had a drill. Lining up at one end of the eight-man blocking sled, we had to hit the first blocking pad, roll, get in a hit the next pad – until all eight were hit. This was not difficult except the other linemen would be hit-roll-hitting right behind you. If you were too slow, the others knocked you over. Those who got knocked over had to run laps.

Now, Coach thought he was improving our speed and reactions. True. But he was also doing something else. He was teaching us *not* to think. Thinking leads to holding back. In a game where an opposing linemen might be heavier and meaner, to hold back and think means a missed or ineffective block and little or no yardage for the ball carrier. It might also mean a trip to the hospital.

A stammerer doing street assignments has the same dynamic as the lightweight offensive guard facing a big mean defensive tackle. Stammerer thinks: 'This person looks grumpy, so I won't ask him.' 'This person looks in a hurry, so I won't ask him.' 'Ah hah! This person looks nice, so I'll ask him.' Too much thinking. Too much holding back. Too much avoiding. This is the central psychological cause of stammering. Here's how to counteract the habit:

Our doubts are traitors, and make us lose the good
we oft might win by fearing to attempt.
WILLIAM SHAKESPEARE

Go to a busy street. Make forty contacts within fifteen minutes. Forty new faces. Make sure your questions can be answered quickly. You should complete a minimum of twenty-five. The record is over 100. Keep at this drill until you get forty.

Now, if you can get forty contacts within fifteen minutes, you can complete 100 within one or two hours. No excuses.

The one-minute hang-up drill

Sometimes it happens. No matter what you do, you just cannot get past the blocks, tricks and avoidances. The prospect of exposing yourself as a stammerer is just too terrifying. You cannot yet concentrate well enough to be fluent in face of the fear. Here's what to do:

Get the yellow pages. Pick out a number. Dial it. Take one minute of mega-severe stammering to ask for yourself. You are to get the person to hang up on you. If the person has not hung up on you after one minute, go from mega-severe to moderately severe stammering and finish your question. Thank them for their patience.

Why should you do this? I will answer this with other questions and answers:

Question: What have you been afraid of all these years?

Answer number 1: You are afraid of being perceived as an out-of-control stammerer.

Answer number 2: You are afraid of someone hanging up or walking away from you.

Question: What is the best remedy for these fears?

Answer: Portraying yourself as a more severe stammerer than you really are and actually trying to get someone to hang up is probably the best way to desensitise you to these fears. Better than hypnosis, better than psychotherapy. You have to do this at least ten times for your fear to come down enough for your concentration to take over. Do not quit just because you did not get immediate results. You will find shortly that the more you try to prolong severe stammering, the more difficult it is to stammer. That terribly agonising one minute will become the incredibly *boring* one minute.

The twenty minute breathing drill
by Allan McGroarty

Among other things, this drill enables you to establish a smooth and continuous motion of the diaphragm and positively returns you to the fundamentals of your physical technique. It involves no speaking. No speaking at all. It does require a commitment of 20 minutes, however.

Sit upright in a comfortable position, preferably in a place where you won't be interrupted, and start your breathing routine. Ensure a full rib expansion on every breath followed by a prolonged push out of air. Make your pauses deliberate – 5 to 10 seconds – before each new inhalation. Keep this routine going continuously for 20 minutes.

This breathing drill will be very familiar to graduates of the McGuire Programme as it is used on McGuire intensive courses, at support meetings and many have adopted it as part of their daily routine. It is repetitive. It is basic stuff. The 20 minute goal forces you past the point of comfort into a zone of concentration and focused effort. There is no escape. 20 minutes. Not 15, not 18, but 20.

Here are the benefits. It allows you to isolate the costal breathing aspect of the McGuire method and concentrate exclusively on that. It reinforces the habit of deliberately pausing, a key factor in speaking well. Practiced regularly, it makes the use of costal breathing during speech more of an automatic response.

There are also some less obvious benefits of the drill. Doing it regularly causes your general anxiety level to come down – deep breathing routines of this kind are often effective as a treatment for panic attacks. Also, people experienced in sport and martial arts training regimes as well as intensive musical instrument practice will recognise that repetitive routines can boost confidence in physical technique and improve concentration.

Note: If you find yourself becoming light-headed, you may be hyperventilating. This is your body's natural reaction to an increase in oxygen. To counter this, stop the breathing drill and hold your breath for a short period. This will retain carbon dioxide in your body and help to restore a proper level of oxygen.

How long? Intensity and persistence.

This process is much like taking an antibiotic when you have some kind of bacterial infection. You have to take the proper dose (intensity), and you have to take it long enough (persistence). If you take two antibiotic pills instead of the prescribed four per day, the bacteria will develop a resistance and the antibiotic won't work. If you stop taking the antibiotic for the prescribed time (because you feel better – see 'Complacency'), the bacteria will develop a resistance and the antibiotic won't work.

If you do not use this method intensely enough, your stammering will develop a resistance and this method will not work.

If you do not use this method long enough, your stammering will develop a resistance and this method will no longer work.

Perhaps the most valuable result of all education
is the ability to make yourself do the thing you have to do,
when it ought to be done, whether you like it or not.
THOMAS HENRY HUXLEY

Contacts: Quantity versus quality

There are times that you need to make many (like hundreds) of short quick contacts to overkill a feared word or sound. Once you have overkilled, however, there is still a need for contacts, but perhaps longer and not so many. Here are some guidelines:

Quantity (many and short contacts)
1. When you have a sticky feared word or sound, you have to take it to the boring stage. This is not negotiable. So far, the only thing that will do this adequately without drug or booze, is many many phone and street contacts starting with the last word that gave you serious trouble. Start easy and work up to more

difficult situations, but go for quantity and get each type of situation to the boring stage before moving on. Then go to the next feared word that gave you trouble, but you will probably find that it doesn't want to play any more after watching you beat up his big buddy. Remember it is that first confrontation with a new face or new voice that will generally bring up the fear.

2. When street contacts are boring no matter what the situation or word, but you still have blocks in real situations. First you have to remind yourself and stand up for your assertive rights of recovery in whatever real situations are giving you the trouble, then you have to do phone and street contacts with whatever word gave you trouble in the situation. It is important, first, to rebuild your confidence, and, second, to see if your blocking has slipped from 'situational' to 'practice'. If you're still 'situational', then ten quick contacts with the word(s) that gave you the trouble in the boring stage should do it for you. This would be 'putting in the wedge' if you were rolling a heavy stone uphill. If, however, you start blocking in 'practice', then you need to follow directions and get down to some heavy overkilling with many many short contacts. Remember, if you are blocking in situations but not in practice, it is most likely an assertiveness problem where you have put the ring back in your nose and forgot that 'you have the right to do whatever is necessary to become a strong, eloquent speaker'.

3. When you need to take 'deliberate dysfluency to the boring stage', if you have any fear of voluntary stammering, then your foundation of 'assertive self acceptance' is rotten and you will constantly relapse.

Warning: Once your feared words and deliberate dysfluency are at the boring stage, *stop* making quantity contacts, as this can be counter-productive as it will use up precious 'juice' that may be needed when you hit more turbulence and need to overkill again.

Quality (fewer but longer contacts)

1. When you've overkilled all feared words to the boring stage, but have some discipline problems, find contacts where you can speak longer, and really focus on technical stuff like long pauses, releasing residual air, good voluntary stammering, etc. Not just have an idle chit chat using sloppy technique.

2. When you feel the need to push out your comfort zone, again, you have already taken feared words and deliberate dysfluency to the boring stage.
3. Testing: everything is great, but you want to see if some historical feared words want to come out and play.

Combat fatigue

Combat soldiers – especially those who have – lost battles or who are entrenched – need breaks. Otherwise they become fatigued and are ineffective as fighters. Occasionally, recovering stammerers will have trouble with phone or street work or both. They continue to grab for tricks no matter how hard they try, or how many situations they go into. Although there is some long-term benefit from simply attacking these situations, it can become counter-productive because tricks and avoidances are being reinforced.

If you are in this rut, drop down to an easier situation such as reading to yourself and practising with friends and family. Do this constantly for a whole day. This means several hours while isolating and exaggerating everything on the checklist – especially deliberate dysfluency. Do several 'hang-up drills'. Then hit the phone and/or streets again the next day with much deliberate dysfluency. You will, however, have to show some guts not to use your tricks and to hit and hold through your blocks if your deliberate dysfluency becomes real.

WARNING: Make an honest attempt to do the regular practice. Do not fall back on the 'combat fatigue' routine without a fight.

> *By perseverance*
> *the snail reached the ark.*
> CHARLES HADDON SPURGEON

The Ratio

Good news and bad news. First the good news: Just doing 100 daily contacts will greatly improve your fluency. Now the bad news: To have any kind of progress, you must (as a minimum) have your words coming through the chest many more times than coming to the mouth. Basic learning theory says that you must 'over learn' the new habit with which you are trying to replace an older habit. To help you do this, graduate and course instructor Heather Lucy composed what we call the:

Ratio Worksheet (by Heather Lucy)

- **Every contact is an opportunity to focus on the various components. Here are some examples:**

RTP	Resist time pressure
RRA	Release residual air
F	Formulate
FP	Focal point
VI	Visualization
P	Pause
FF	Fast and Full
Q	Quiet in the chest
PT	Perfect timing
AFS	Assertive first sound
KMF	Keep moving forward
DBT	Deep breathy tone
A	Articulation
DD	Deliberate Dysfluency
BR	Block release
HH	Hit and hold

- Decide, <u>before</u> starting your contact session, which items you are going to focus on. Fill in the top row of the Contact Ratio Worksheet with your chosen items, (or complete the already prepared one).
- Decide, <u>before</u> doing an individual contact, which <u>specific item</u> you are going to focus on.

<u>After</u> each contact record your own evaluation by filling in the appropriate box with either:

+	Full and correct use of the method
I	Room for improvement e.g. speaking process came up to your mouth, using a trick, filler word, avoiding or substituting.

- **Remember EVERY contact is a success.**

    The + contacts: pat yourself on the back – exciting

    The I contacts: are an opportunity to learn – exciting

- **Look at your ratio of + : I**

    Is it better than your last contact session?

    30 : 70,   60 : 40,   80 : 20,   95 : 5,   100 : 0   How are you doing?

    Are you pleased with your progress, if so congratulate yourself.

- **Make a note of challenging words and keep challenging them!**

Remember, you still need to continuously keep to **The Laws** (Chapter 9)

100 Contacts Ratio Worksheet   **Date:**

Item	RRA	DBT	AFS	FF	RTP	DD	BR	HH		
1										
2										
3										
4										
5										
6										
7										
8										
9										
10										

Challenging words:	Number of + is
	Number of I is
	Ratio of + : I is

Make several copies of this worksheet and put together a "workbook". Then . . . go to work!

CHAPTER SEVEN:

Battle-hardened – tournament tough

Our greatest glory consists not of ever falling,
but in rising every time we fall.
RALPH WALDO EMERSON

So you've drilled this new speaking technique until you are doing it in your sleep. And you've drilled your non-avoidance so much in the streets and on the phone that the police are looking for you. Now it's time to kill the monster. It is time to destroy his home.

A young recruit enters a Marine Corps boot camp. In this Rite of Passage, he is mentally and physically broken down and transformed from fun-loving teenager to killer. He is issued a weapon and is trained how to use it. He participates in war games to practise using his weapon and tactics in battlefield conditions.

This is the true joy in life, the being used for a
purpose recognised by yourself as a mighty one; the
being thoroughly worn out before you are thrown on
the scrap heap; the being a force of nature instead of
a feverish selfish little clod of ailments and
grievances complaining that the world will not
devote itself to making you happy.
GEORGE BERNARD SHAW

He is not, however, a dependable soldier. He must now become **battle-hardened**. The only way to become battle-hardened is in combat. He must test his courage by facing death.

A general will battle-harden raw recruits by throwing them into a less important battle. Some military historians say that is why the untested American army first fought the superior German army in North Africa. The goal wasn't winning or losing, but to develop a core of combat veterans for more critical battles.

The sports analogy

It's one thing for a tennis player to hold on to his technique and game plan in a friendly match. It is quite another to do this in formal competition where winning or losing takes on a new dimension. Especially if you are on a team where your matches mean the difference between the team winning or losing. Muscles tighten. Thinking fogs. Here comes that easy lob. You hit the ball against the back fence. You never miss such a shot in a friendly match.

> *Winning can be defined*
> *as the science of being totally prepared.*
> GEORGE ALLEN (1902–89)

So formal competition is a different game. There is definitely a punishment for losing, and there is definitely a reward for winning. It is life's process wrapped up in a few hours. It is doubtful that immediate execution of the loser by firing squad would produce greater intensity. Even at the beginning level a certain amount of life and death is involved. The life or death of one's self-esteem. For a healthy person this 'death' is just a fleeting, half-second feeling. For an unhealthy person, the demoralisation can last for days: it is much more than a stupid game.

A tennis player wants at least to play well in competition. At least to give his opponent a good match – to play well in formal competition – a tennis player must become 'tournament tough'. How does one become tournament tough? PLAY A LOT OF TOURNAMENTS!

And just like the general throwing untested soldiers into unimportant battles in preparation for important ones, a tennis player will enter smaller tournaments in preparation for the bigger ones.

Recovering stammerers also need to become battle-hardened tournament tough. Street and telephone drills are great for practising your technique, assertiveness, and can reduce fear. They are like war games for soldiers and practice matches for tournament tennis players. But these are not the real battles. They are not real tournaments.

Real speaking battles are the core of your iceberg. Speaking tournaments have a consequence for your stammering going out of control or reward for reasonable fluency. People who you will never have to deal with again have no substantial reward or punishment. What are real battle/tournament situations? Things like:

- In-laws (or prospective in-laws) are real battle/tournament situations.
- Potential love relationships are real battle/tournament situations.
- Job interviews are real battle/tournament situations.
- Speaking with your boss is a real battle/tournament situation.
- Speaking in class.
- Oral presentations at work.

These speaking situations are the 'big battles', the grand-slam tournaments. You cannot stay in the trenches or clubhouse. You must prepare for these battles/tournaments and attack them. You cannot wait for these situations to come to you. You must seek them out. You do not wait for your boss to call you into his office – you call him for an appointment to speak to him (about anything). You do not wait for your mother-in-law to call you – you call her.

How do you prepare for major battles/tournaments? Answer: find a less stressful but similar individual situation. You must do some creative thinking, but here are some suggestions:

Arrange to speak to the mothers of some friends before contact with your mother-in-law.

> *Don't let life discourage you; everyone who got where he is*
> *had to begin where he was.*
> RICHARD L. EVANS

Arrange some job interviews even though you have no intention of taking the position offered. Get accustomed to speaking to someone who has the power to hire and fire before you deal with the person who indeed has this power over you.

Practise speaking before groups by joining and attending speaker's clubs such as Toastmasters. This will help you become eloquent. You can find one through telephone information, the library, universities, etc. Locating one is good practice. If there is no speaker's club in your area, start one. It is a simple matter of placing an advertisement in local newspapers, sending letters out to companies, putting notices on bulletin boards. Toastmasters will send you guidelines for starting a chapter and running meetings.

Take a foreign language class. Although you will eventually be called to speak, you must volunteer to speak. Speaking in a foreign language is extremely good for your fluency as it requires more time during the pause (therefore more time-pressure resistance) to translate as well as formulate. Becoming fluent in a foreign language is part of becoming eloquent. It is fun, especially when you visit that foreign country.

Warming up

Say you show up two hours early for the Wimbledon finals. As you are walking around looking in the shops to kill time before the match starts, what do you think Agassi and Sampras are doing? Watching cartoons in the players' lounge? No. They are on the back practice courts drilling forehands, backhands, volleys, overheads, serves, returns, etc. Then they spend some time just thinking and rehearsing their game plans. They might have a five-set match ahead of them, but they will still be out on the practice court for an hour. Why? Because it is important that every component of their games is 'tuned' before the points start counting.

> *Before everything else,*
> *Getting ready is the secret of success.*
> HENRY FORD (1863–1947)

You, too, need to warm up before difficult speaking situations. This includes practising the components of your checklist. It also includes knowing your subject matter (as much as possible) and how you are going to present it so that you don't get caught in the 'competence vs. incompetence' approach-avoidance conflict. It includes giving yourself some quiet time before the situation to centre yourself with some diaphragm meditation.

Regrouping

After the British were badly defeated in Western Europe, they evacuated their troops from Dunkirk and regrouped to fight again. After the Soviets were badly defeated during Hitler's Operation Barbarossa, they moved their weapons factories beyond the Urals and regrouped to fight again.

You might lose some battles in this war against the oppression of stammering. You'll be in an important meeting or interview and will experience a chest freezer that will lead to another and another and another until you are grabbing uncontrollably for your old tricks and avoiding words. If you have been sailing on automatic for a while, it is probably too late to stammer voluntarily, image, focus, etc. This stuff must be practised regularly if you want it to work in those surprise situations – but we all get lazy and overconfident.

The best thing to do in such a situation is be honest. Ask for a break, 'Excuse me. I've been recovering from stammering and I'm having a relapse. Please give me a few minutes to get myself together.' Just acknowledging your role as a stammerer will take away much of the pressure – after all, your tricks and avoidances are just ways to hide this fact. Two circles start to overlap . . . stress comes down.

If you can get a short break from the situation, do strong costal breathing with long pauses. Force yourself to image the diaphragm in your thorax. Remind yourself again to feel your voice coming deeply through your chest. Remember: the basic goal of this whole programme is to get your speaking process down in your chest and fluency becomes the by-product.

If your stammering is still out-of-control after this, try to shut up. If you are stuck in the speaking situation, just do the best you can. As the German army in the Battle of the Bulge, your dying stammering monster has broken through your line of defence. You will need to acknowledge that this battle has been lost. You must regroup, retrain, call in reinforcements and counter-attack. Get your Ratio Worksheet, get on the telephone, go out in the streets, find another similar (but less important) situation and attack.

Good news and bad news: The good news is that, if you react immediately and intensely, your counterattacks will be successful and you will win the war. The bad news is that, if you do not regroup immediately and intensely, your counter-attack will fail and you will lose the war.

> *What counts is not necessarily the size of the dog in the fight –*
> *it's the size of the fight in the dog.*
> DWIGHT D. EISENHOWER

CHAPTER EIGHT:

Crisis management

What to do when things fall apart

*Obstacles are things a person sees
when he takes his eyes off his goal.*
JOSEPH E. COSSMAN

So you've been flying high on automatic for weeks, months or even years. You thought the shame, guilt, self-hate and panic was dead and buried . . . a thing of the past never to return. **Then it happens:**

Suddenly (probably a day when everything else is going wrong and your hexagon is screwed up mega in the negative) it hits you. Perhaps it is something about the person behind the counter. Or something about the store's decorations. Or the colour of the hair of the person standing behind you. Who knows what will trigger it: probably a combination of stimuli, that includes your current state of mind.

Before you know it, those old feelings of terror well up from your subconscious. The old 'I'm not going to be able to get this word out'. You and your diaphragm go into a giant approach-avoidance conflict and you have a nasty block known in the McGuire Programme as a '**chest freezer**'.

But that's not the end of it. In spite of the warning that this would happen, the terror feelings are followed closely by feelings of discouragement and despair. Old tapes start again: 'Nothing I do will get the word out.' 'This method isn't working and will never work.' 'My stammering is going out of control.' And so forth. *So what happened?*

Most likely (before the crisis) you had let yourself go back to speaking from the crural diaphragm while you were enjoying your automatic fluent speech. After all, non-stammerers always speak from the crural diaphragm. When the fear hit, your crural diaphragm went into its chronic contractions and it was too late to engage the costal diaphragm in the face of the surprise element, which led to panic. Then, although we have no scientific research to support this, maybe your lower brain couldn't decide between using the costal or the crural diaphragm, so it short-circuited the phrenic nerve. (Or something like that.) Then that seemingly living nasty entity we call 'stammering' brings up its reinforcements:

Despair

Think back to when you had tried everything to get words out. Remember the hopeless 'No matter what I do, I can't stop stammering'. I, personally, remember the endless hours of reading out loud at night, hoping that it would help me be fluent the next day – but it never worked, even though I gave it my absolute best shot. *Webster's Dictionary* defines despair as 'utter loss of hope'. Hopelessness. After so many experiences of these thoughts of hopelessness, it is small wonder that they remain even after we've reached automatic (even eloquent) fluency.

There was a study done which verified that punishment-based learning is irreversible. And stammering is most definitely punishment-based learning. You were punished (in some way) every time you stammered. And the punishment strengthened the stammering by strengthening the avoidance reaction. So it is possibly true that stammering is not totally curable – but don't let this be an excuse not to work and fight.

So the feelings of 'nothing I do will help' will possibly be with you indefinitely. And they will come bursting forth like a visit from an unemployed relative with every block. The best thing to do is to realise that these feelings are just old tapes and TAKE ACTION.

> *Courage is the price that life exacts for granting peace.*
> *The soul that knows it not, knows no release*
> *From little things;*
> *Knows not the livid loneliness of fear,*
> *Nor mountain highs where bitter joy can hear*
> *The sound of wings.*
> AMELIA EARHART

Now, say you have experienced a relapse where you are once again mired in the swamp of tricks and avoidance. You had felt free but, like a bird in an oil slick, you are now having a very difficult time taking off again. You start your blast-off routine again. You put six hours and 300 situations in one day. You go to bed improved, but still blocking badly. The tendency is to quit. Don't. Let me explain what is happening:

Any athlete or musician who is facing a tough competition or performance after a long lay-off experiences the exact same thing. In my tennis days I would not practise during the winter. Then in April the outdoor clay courts would open and inter-club competition would begin. (Competition between clubs is the high point of Dutch tennis with significant money going to players in the top classes.) On the first practice day I could barely hit a decent backhand, much less do well in a competitive match. At some point came the feeling, 'I am a bad tennis player – I will never get my game back'. But I would keep trying. The next day I would drag my body on to the court against the current of negative thoughts that scream: 'I hate tennis – why do I bother?' But amazingly, there would be a considerable improvement. Something had happened during sleep to bring back my skills. On the third day, my old game would return.

Trying to recover your fluency after a bad fall will follow this pattern. The first day of practice will be discouraging. But if you push yourself and do your best, the second day should be much better. By the third or fourth day your high-point should be back – even stronger, because you proved to yourself that you could indeed recover relatively quickly from a relapse.

The spot of rust, the messy house, the pound of fat

Rust

Your car is being eaten away by rust. Big holes forming around the windows and under the doors. You take your rusty wheels to a body shop. The rust is sanded off, holes filled, anti-rust compound applied. Then the car is repainted and looks like new again.

Months later a spot of rust again appears. Not surprising as rust tends to have the same characteristics as cancer. If the spot of rust is not taken care of (sanded, anti-rust compound, new paint) it will quickly metastasise and your car will need another expensive trip to the body shop (or the junk yard) which could have been prevented if you had taken care of the rust when it was a little spot.

The mess

My wife and I should have an award for being the world's messiest housekeepers. We both had sweet mothers who cleaned our rooms because they wanted us to have time to do other productive things. So we never developed the habit of picking up after ourselves. Add to this two messy children and you have a certified disaster area. We have a cleaning lady who comes in once a month. She keeps asking for more money because our house is 'special'. After she works all morning, the house is actually presentable. One hour later, however, it has returned its original condition. Every so often I attempt to reverse this pattern. It is like a religious experience. The neighbours know it when they hear a certain scream coming from the McGuire establishment. I go through the house throwing everything not in its proper place in a bag. Then I dump everything in the big toy box muttering 'If they want it, they'll have to dig around until they find it'. This includes my wife's handbag and jewellery. Then I give them THE LAW:

ALL FLAT SURFACES MUST BE EMPTY. ANYTHING FOUND OUT OF PLACE WILL BE DUMPED!

It is amazing how good a house looks when there is nothing on the counters, tables, floors. Just a couple of crying kids who can't find their Barbies. 'A place for everything and everything in its place,' my father always said. Then it happens: the half-eaten sandwich on the piano. The baseball glove on the table. The dirty socks on the couch. Like cancer cells, these quickly metastasise into an uncontrolled, overwhelming mess. In a few months the neighbours again hear 'the scream' from the McGuire house.

Fat

I have a fat problem. It started back when I wanted to play college football. A 160-pound defensive end didn't have much of a chance in college. I needed to put on weight. Every night I went to the weight room. I also needed to eat more. Problem was, I was poor. Food costs money. So I got a job in the cafeteria. Every time the supervising cook wasn't looking, I stuffed my face. I remember the hard-boiled eggs. The chunks of pastrami. The bread rolls. Everything and anything. Not that far removed from John Belushi in his famous cafeteria scene in the movie *Animal House*.

So I quickly went from 160 to 200 pounds. But I couldn't lift weights fast enough (and study) to keep the fat off. Many fat cells were created. Although these shrunk when I later lost weight, they were always there waiting for the chance to fill up again. Every time my lifestyle changed to where I was not getting enough exercise, I got fat.

The pattern is always the same. The first extra pound. The second extra pound. The old 'I should go running now but I'm too tired.' The old 'I shouldn't eat this, but I deserve it because I've worked so hard – I need to replenish my energy . . .' Soon, my size 34 shorts and underwear are at the bottom of my wardrobe, and I am shopping for size 36 – swearing that 36 is the absolute limit.

It would have been *so* much easier if I would have taken care of those first few pounds immediately. Now I face dealing with at least 20 pounds of stubborn fat. Either another three month juice fast, or a slow painful diet both followed by a commitment to change my lifestyle and include more exercise. At this point, however, I think I will go to my grave in my size 36 undees . . . but my last words will have been fluent.

(Bad) habits gather by unseen degrees,
As brooks make rivers,
Rivers run to seas.
JOHN DRYDEN (1631–1700)

Take care of that first little spot of rust immediately and you don't have to take your car to the body shop. Take care of the half-eaten sandwich on the piano immediately and you can keep your house presentable. Take care of that first extra pound immediately and you don't have to go through another major diet.

So what is that first spot of rust? The answer is simple: it is a word. Of course! It is a stupid *word* which brings the fear, followed by panic, followed by the block followed (or preceded) perhaps by a trick or avoidance. And this word probably starts with a sound which in your dark stammering past caused you the most trouble. More than likely it was a word which started with the first sound of your name.

TAKE CARE OF THAT FIRST WORD WHERE YOU BLOCKED, USED A TRICK AND/OR AVOIDED AND YOUR STAMMERING WON T GO OUT OF CONTROL.

The return of your stammering is not the result of some mysterious, incomprehensible demonic force. It follows the same laws as rusty cars, fat bodies, messy houses. *You* can maintain your fluency. Or *you* can go back to being a verbal cripple.

The Battle of the 'Dit'

I had been totally fluent for several months. Perhaps only a few little reminders, but nothing that threatened my precious fluency. Then it happened. I was trying to convince someone to buy one tennis string for his racquet rather than the other. In Dutch it was 'dit snaar is beter dan de andere.' Maybe it was because I wasn't being 100 per cent honest (there was very little difference between the two strings.) Or maybe my time was up. Or maybe because I wasn't sure if the proper Dutch word was 'deze' or 'dit' which caused another approach-avoidance conflict. Whatever the cause, I seriously blocked on 'dit'. Much more than a 'little reminder'. When the customer left, I went to the phone and said 'dit is Dave McGuire . . . etc.' After five blocks in a row, I saw visions of going back to slavery not to mention closing my Institute. The fear became intense, but I kept fighting. Finally it started coming deep out of my chest. I did about thirty extra phone calls, each time beginning with 'dit' to make sure. Whenever the phone rang, I answered it with 'dit is Dave McGuire' rather than the usual 'Dave McGuire'. I went to bed relieved that I had got it back.

Diamonds are nothing more than chunks of coal
that stuck to their jobs.
MALCOLM FORBES

The next morning, however, I had another block on the same word. But I got it back down in my chest quicker this time and it stayed down for the rest of the day.

The third day, I had one or two mild blocks in the morning. I went into every stressful situation I could find using 'dit'. No blocks, no tricks. The three-day Battle of the Dit was over. I still felt fear when the phone rang, but the fear subsided after several times, proving that I could indeed keep it down deep in the face of fear.

As with the Battle of the Bulge, it was a close call. **It started with a stupid three-letter word**. Had I not dealt with it effectively as I did, it would have spread to all 'd' words. Then to all hard sounds. Very soon, I would have had to close the Freedom's Road programme. Because I won, others have won.

What can you learn from this? Several things:

1. **Know the initial word that gave you trouble. In a feared situation, you might have blocked on several words, but it always starts with** ONE **word.**

2. **Respond immediately to this word. Do not procrastinate. If you go to bed that night without having given it your best effort, the problem will magnify the next day.**

3. **Keep pounding intensely at this word. It may take you days to kill the panic surrounding this word, but the fighting will keep it from metastasising to other words. If you are half-hearted, the problem will increase. Be able to look yourself in the mirror every night and say, 'I did my best. I fought my hardest.'**

4. **Do not quit. You may not recover the first day. It might even take you a lot of intense fighting. You will experience despair and discouragement, but don't let this be an excuse to stop fighting.**

5. **Dig up your 'Ratio Worksheets'. Use them.**

> **6.** **If you get stuck several times on a feared word where you grab for tricks to avoid, drop down to a less feared situation to practise. Then hit it again in the more feared situations. But don't stay in the trenches too long cleaning your weapon in an effort to postpone the attack while the enemy's tanks are rolling over you.**
>
> **7. Go back and review 'Overkill' in Chapter Three.**

The Slippery Slope

Recovery from stammering usually follows an exponential curve upwards. Progress is slow at first then, if one works hard and follows directions, improvement is increasingly rapid.

Relapse also follows this exponential pattern. Regression is at first imperceptible, but (with increasing use of tricks and avoidance) quickly becomes a free-fall. If response is inadequate, you crash and burn. Then you have to start all over again.

Good news and bad news: The good news is that, if you take care of those first few feared words, you will quickly get your fluency back. Your fluency will probably be stronger when you have proved to yourself that you can indeed get it back. The bad news is, if you don't take care of those words, the problem will metastasise and you will have a relapse.

Spin pull-out

So – regardless of the warnings – you let yourself get away with those first few tricks and avoidance. You are in a free-fall. You can barely speak a fluent word with your dog. The same thing happens to pilots. It is called a spin.

Back in my stammering days I took flying lessons but quit because of one too many blocks on the radio. The approach-avoidance dynamics of my stammering also tended to make me freeze during take-offs and landings. My instructor was getting nervous. But I learned something about spin recovery.

An aeroplane has to keep a smooth flow of air over the wings in order to stay in the air. If (because of too steep a climb, turbulence, etc.,) this airflow is disrupted, the aeroplane goes into a 'stall', followed quickly by a downward spin.

Student pilots are trained to put their aeroplanes into a stall on purpose, so that they can practise pulling out of spin. The idea is to fly out of the spin. This means one must put nose down, put the throttle forward, and turn (still nose down) in the direction of the spin.

At first it is terrifying for the student pilot. If unsuccessful, he will die. But after a few successful pull-outs, however, the student realises he can do it every time. Then recovery from spins becomes fun.

But there's a catch: To recover from a spin, a student pilot must respond quickly and intensely. There is not a whole lot of time to be slow and lazy.

And of course, recovery from a spin is assuming the aeroplane has enough altitude. Which is why one must keep the throttle forward during takeoffs and why one must be very careful during landings.

So what are the parallels to stammering? Should be obvious, but I will spell them out:

The stall

If a pilot responds immediately to a stall, he will not go into a spin. If a recovering stammerer responds immediately to that first feared word, trick or avoidance, he will not relapse.

The spin

Sometimes spins and relapses happen. If a pilot responds immediately and intensely (nose down, full throttle) to a spin, he will easily recover if he has enough altitude and doesn't panic when he realises he must go down before he can go up. If a recovering stammerer responds immediately and intensely to a severe relapse, he too will recover if he has enough altitude and doesn't panic.

The crash

The pilot will die if he can't pull out of his spin. You will not die if you can't pull out of your stammering spin. You will just have to face the demoralisation of having to start all over again.

On page 120 is the 'Spin pull-out checklist'. Use this as a guideline and evaluation of your response to relapse.

The Forest Fire

In 1985, I spent some time fighting a forest fire. Fighting a forest fire is about the closest thing to war one can experience. Like an infantryman in the rear trenches, I recall sitting in a fire truck half asleep watching battalions of soldiers – with their 'weapons' of shovels, axes, and chain saws – move up to the front line. Each fire fighting company had its own uniforms with special emblems for the elite units of proven veterans. I could see the glow of the fire over the ridge and hear its faint roar. There was the roar, too, of water bombers. The driver, much experienced in this warfare, warned me that, should the wind shift, we could be fighting for our lives. In the meantime, our biggest job was staying awake.

The next day, groggy from forty-eight hours of no sleep, we went to the battlefield. Fresh troops were still moving up to the fire line that had moved on. Our job was to 'mop up' the hot spots. Looking over the burned area, I could see small wisps of smoke rising from certain places. Occasionally, there would be a red glow or even a flame.

The experienced fighters showed me what to do. Dragging the heavy hose from the tanker truck, every suspected spot had to be dug up, doused with water, chopped up, doused again, turned, doused again. One would think that just a good turning and a little water would be sufficient. But it wasn't. There was still much burnable fuel on the ground plus dry areas that the original fire had missed. If these hot spots weren't completely extinguished another major fire could flare up again. Then a wind shift could set alight the unburned areas, trapping firefighters who were battling the main blaze.

Same with you after pulling out of a bad relapse. You need to dig up every possible feared word or feared situation, douse it with every aspect of this method including deliberate dysfluency, chop it up, douse it again.

Spin pull-out checklist

In this journey to fluency's freedom, we all hit 'turbulence' where we lose confidence. If you do not react quickly and intensely enough, this leads to a fall where your stammering will go out of control. The following is to help you evaluate your response to this relapse spin. Those who have not experienced such a fall should predict their response. Are you, have you been, or will you be:

1. Cancelling every trick and avoidance?
2. Deliberate dysfluency at least once per two breaths?
3. Using a belt to help with your rib expansion?
4. Taking at least two costal breaths per minute during waking hours with pause, full inhale, full rib expansion?
5. Using the basic method with everything you say?
6. Dedicating at least two hours a day to practise (outside school and work) until you pull out of your spin and become stronger than you were before?
7. Increasing, if necessary, your practice time?
8. Getting up an hour earlier and going to bed an hour later, if necessary, to put in extra practice time?
9. Starting every morning with phone calls to practise partners if you have one?
10. Buying, reading, and utilising all recommended books?
11. Taking responsibility for your difficulties (as opposed to finding excuses)?
12. Aggressively seeking out speaking situations?
13. Doing your best to resist the temptation to use tricks and avoid?
14. Practising imaging the diaphragm or holding a focal point as part of your practice and whenever possible during waking hours?
15. Willing to give up alcohol and/or drugs if they are (even possibly) interfering with your recovery?
16. Using the Yellow Pages, classified newspaper adverts, and other adverts?
17. Doing morning and bedtime breathing exercises?
18. Completing at least one 'Ratio Worksheet' every day?
19. Responding immediately and intensely to severe turbulence?

20. Going regularly to a Speakers' Club and/or foreign language class?
21. Sticking with the winners (those who will help motivate you to work harder as opposed to those who help you find excuses)?
22. Actively preparing and planning to attack your remaining feared situations?
23. At least three 'hang-up calls' per day?

Counting the number of times you answered 'yes', here's how to evaluate yourself:

- A score of 20 to 25 indicates that you either have had no significant relapses or have had only a few from which you quickly recovered.
- A score of 16 to 20 indicates that you probably had a severe relapse, have recovered, but could have recovered quicker and stronger.
- A score of 12 to 16 indicates that you have probably had several relapses from which you've never really recovered to a high fluency. You are in danger of falling into the chronic relapse pattern.
- A score 8 to 12 indicates you chronically bounce from less-than-satisfactory fluency to out-of-control stammering. You are not really improving. Your effort to improve is inadequate. You have fallen into a chronic relapse pattern and are in danger of giving up. A change of attitude as shown in increased intensity and work will allow you to improve and eventually reach freedom. Be aware that you will now have to work harder than someone who is has not fallen into this pattern because you have to deal with 'the fear of another severe relapse' on top of the fear of stammering and fear of losing your fluency.
- A score below 8 indicates that it's time for you do a major attitude adjustment or stop wasting your time with this method. Another stammering programme might be beneficial.

CHAPTER NINE:

How to lose it

Last night at twelve I felt immense,
But now I feel like thirty cents.
GEORGE ADE (1902)

The Laws

'Look at any stutterer who is still stuttering severely or has relapsed and you see someone who has cheated on the principle of avoidance reduction.' Dr J. Sheehan

There are indeed laws governing stammering, which are as unyielding as the laws of physics and chemistry. Unlike as with social laws, the punishment for breaking these laws is fixed: you will continue to stammer uncontrollably, you will relapse, you will never reach freedom. There is no probation or suspended sentences. You will always have to pay the fine and/or go to jail. But what are these laws? Looking at what has caused me to start blocking again, here are eight:

LAW NUMBER ONE: *Do not use tricks*
You should know what tricks are by now. Old ones will keep trying to come back. New ones will try to develop. Be aware that tricks work wonderfully well when you've been 'clean' for a while. As with drugs and booze, however, tricks are a sure way to relapse. Don't fool yourself. You will never recover and you will always relapse if you continue to use tricks.

*The problem is not that there are problems. The problem is
expecting otherwise, and thinking that
having problems is a problem.*
THEODORE RUBIN

LAW NUMBER TWO: *Do not avoid words or sounds*
Substituting a feared word with a non-feared word or a feared syllable will elicit more fear than tricks. You will never reach fluency if you continue to avoid words or sounds. You will always relapse if you continue to avoid words or sounds.

We must travel in the direction of our fear
JOHN BERRYMAN (1914–72) A POINT OF AGE

LAW NUMBER THREE: *Do not avoid situations*
You may not be fluent when a television reporter sticks a microphone in your face, but you must try. You might even use tricks in such a tough situation, but it is better than running away. Consciously avoiding a situation will increase your fear more than anything.

If you do go into a tough situation and have many blocks, avoid words and use tricks, make firm plans and preparations to go back into this or a similar situation. This is like a tennis player, who gets beaten badly in a tournament, and who increases and intensifies his practice sessions, then signs up for and plays in another tournament. He may get beaten again, but he repeats this process until he rises to a higher level. He may never reach Wimbledon, but he will at least reach his potential. He will at least be a competent tennis player as you can be a competent speaker.

LAW NUMBER FOUR: *Immediately cancel violations of the above laws*
This is your 'fine'. The habits formed by punishment-based learning are very tenacious. And stammering's tricks and avoidance are most definitely the result of punishment-based learning – tricks and avoidance are a response to fear. Therefore, even the strongest ex-stammerer will experience those surprise situations, which will elicit a block which, in turn, elicits an avoidance mechanism.

Unless one is more than human, this will probably happen several times during recovery. You can forgive yourself for it.

He that diggeth a pit shall fall into it.
ECCLESIASTES: 10.8

You cannot, however, forgive yourself for *not* cancelling every trick or avoidance. And you must do it before you go to bed. You can pay a small fine now, or wait and go to jail. If you do not cancel a trick or avoidance, this habit will be stronger and you will continue to use tricks and avoid. If you do not cancel your tricks and avoiding, you will never reach freedom. You will always relapse.

LAW NUMBER FIVE: *Put in whatever effort is necessary*
You need to put out a certain amount of time and energy to recover. If you are not improving, then you must increase your efforts until you do. Once you've broken free of stammering's gravitational pull (orbit zone) you can stay there with minimum effort. But until you break free, you must invest time and energy. You cannot be lazy.

There are no shortcuts
to any place worth going.
ANON

If you are into a steep relapse spin or have crashed, you must do everything on the turbulence checklist. If you cannot get yourself going, you must return to an intensive course/refresher ASAP. If you do not respond intensively, you will never reach freedom. You will always relapse.

LAW NUMBER SIX: *Respond immediately to turbulence*
Sometimes you will hit some situations, which elicit a deal of fear. Especially if you deal with this fear with tricks and avoidance, you will quickly begin to relapse. The longer you wait to respond, the further you will have to climb back and continue your flight to freedom. Immediate response to turbulence must become a habit. If you continue to procrastinate your responses to turbulence, this procrastination will become a habit. If pro-

crastination becomes a habit, you will never reach freedom. You will always relapse.

> *Fall seven times, stand up eight.*
> JAPANESE PROVERB

LAW NUMBER SEVEN: Respond intensely to turbulence

If you respond to turbulence with an inadequate effort, you will continue to fall. The further you fall, the further you have to climb back. You must develop the habit of responding intensely to turbulence and relapse spins. If inadequate responses become a habit, you will never reach freedom. You will always have severe relapses.

> *It is no use saying, 'We are doing our best'.*
> *You have got to succeed in doing what is necessary.*
> WINSTON CHURCHILL.

LAW NUMBER EIGHT: Your response to turbulence must be long enough

If you quit your intense response to turbulence too soon, you will never reach freedom. You will always have severe relapses. You will eventually reach your previous level of stammering.

> *You can let yourself off the hook,*
> *but the laws governing stuttering will never let you off the hook.*
> DR J. SHEEHAN

Mechanisms of failure

What do we need to obey the above laws? What do you need to go beyond stuttering to eloquence and hold on to it? Two things:

Work Ethic (including perseverance) to put in the work necessary to get good.

Courage to push out their comfort zones, face their feared situations, and take reasonable risks.

You can fail to get what you want or lose it once you got it with the same mechanisms that anyone will manipulate himself or herself into not reaching or losing their goals. If we dive deeper into this, there are some other personality traits, 'mechanisms', or habitual behaviours, that promote and maintain less than satisfactory work ethic and/or courage. I've pinpointed five, but maybe there are more:

Arrogance

You think you're too cool, intelligent, educated, rich, etc. to follow directions and work hard. Maybe you think you're smarter than your coach, know more about stammering than the guy writing this book, make more money, drive a fancy car, live in a big house, younger, better looking, etc. Arrogance could be seen as the root of the following four traps.

> *When they discover the centre of the universe,*
> *a lot of people will be disappointed*
> *to discover they are not it.*
> BERNARD BAILEY

Denial

Almost everyone has heard of this before. Nothing new. An athlete will deny the fact that skipping practice or getting drunk the night before a game will negatively affect performance. An alcoholic about to come off the wagon will deny the fact that taking that one drink will put him right back in the gutter. A person trying to overcome stammering will deny the fact that using tricks and avoiding words will cause more severe stammering. All are discounting or denying that the problem is really all that bad or that they are regressing. On another level, the whole game of stammering revolves around denial and lying. I avoided words and situations and used tricks in an attempt to deny that I was a stammerer and to lie that I was a fluent speaker. It is small wonder that denial and lying carries over to other things the biggest of which is denying that stammering is indeed a BIG problem.

The alcoholic denies that a few drinks are really dangerous to their recovery from alcoholism. The stammerer denies that tricks and avoidance are really damaging to fluency or progress towards fluency.

Complacency
'This is good enough', 'I'm a lot better than I was before' is the message you give to yourself. You forgot that being good at anything means continuing to improve. Someone trying to lose weight will think: 'Well, I've lost ten pounds. I deserve that googoo pie.' Of course, denial plays a role in this.

Intellectualisation
You do your homework to find arguments against doing what needs to be done to get what you want; arguing definitions and concepts; challenging basic philosophies of the programme and which rationale is valid instead of addressing the issue directly. Naturally you do this because you're smart, or think you're smart. (Arrogant?) Intellectualisers are constantly outsmarting themselves. If they would put the same effort into just following directions rather than research excuses to be lazy and not brave, they just might make some significant improvement.

> *Knowing is not enough; we must apply.*
> *Willing is not enough;*
> *we must do.*
> GOETHE

Commonly heard stuff from those who engage in too much intellectualisation:

'What is addiction/trick-using really?' 'Is tightening up my mouth really a trick?' 'Is speaking fast really a trick?'

'This other (famous) programme I was in uses syllabic/blended contact speech/etc., so it can't be a trick.'

'This (recovery from stammering) is not really like sport.'

'It is simply not practical (fair and reasonable) to put this amount of time and effort into this.'

'Deliberate dysfluency brings back my real blocks, therefore, this is not a valid technique, therefore I won't do it.'

'I heard so-and-so (who was recovered) have some big blocks. Therefore this technique is not valid (therefore I can alter it – incorporate tricks.)'

Externalisation

This is the no-brainer's intellectualisation. You simply blame someone else or something else for not getting what you want. Easy. Key word is 'responsibility' . . . not taking enough of it for your own mistakes and failures.

So okay. We all do these things at one point or another. It's when you do it too much so that too many things you want are not becoming realities that it's time to step back and take a look at yourself and what you're doing.

What to do about it? It's not rocket science. Just habits that need to be replaced with better, more productive habits. Build your character. Know these traps so that you can recognise them every time you feel yourself using these 'tools' to be lazy when you need to work, and cowardly when you need to be brave.

Other things that keep us from getting what we want

If the above are the tools that lead to working not so hard as we should, or being not so brave as we should, here are some personality traits that, if you have too much of these, can keep you from making the progress you want, even if you are working hard and being brave. It is beyond the scope of this book to solve these for you, but there are many self-help books around as well as effective growth workshops and therapists.

Too much stress

We all know what stress is. Those who study it say it is caused by the classic 'flight or fight' response to danger. Sounds like an approach-avoidance conflict to me. Approach-avoidance conflicts in one part of your life will lead to the fear-of-stammering approach-avoidance conflict. For the substance abuser, it becomes an excuse to start his/her drug use again. For the recovering stammerer, it becomes an excuse to start avoiding and using tricks again. Or to stop working.

A person trying to overcome stammering is already under a great deal of stress simply from the recovery process. And stress has a direct connection to the diaphragm. There isn't a lot of room for stress from other sources such as relationships, money, etc.

Here are some aggravators of stress:

Perfectionism

Perhaps you see another stammerer who has attained fluency. You want to be totally fluent in every situation and you want it now. Not getting it now (or within your unrealistic deadline) or a surprise block triggers the stress reaction. Of course, this goes right to your diaphragm and slows your recovery.

Then you start looking for – and finding – excuses for why it's not working faster and more perfectly for you. This takes away from the concentration and effort required to reach eloquence. So your progress is even slower. You're in danger of throwing everything out of the window and grab for your tricks and avoidance. Of course you'll have a 'good, valid' excuse for doing so.

A big part of perfectionism is wanting to be the star. The 'If I can't be on the first team, I quit (this is a crappy team anyway)' syndrome. Those who go faster than you probably have reduced their iceberg of feared situations more than you – probably because they did more non-avoidance training than you. Or maybe because they have spent more time developing their powers of concentration. And they are probably recovering faster than you because they are not dealing with the stress of perfectionism.

Low frustration tolerance

You fall apart under pressure. Any time you experience fear in a situation, you grab for tricks. You probably have great difficulty holding a focal point or diaphragm image for any length of time. As with perfectionism, you are in danger of throwing the whole method out of the window.

Excessive worrying

We all know about worrying. Sitting around thinking if something you did was bad, or if something you're about to do will be bad or good. Not taking action to resolve your doubts. Wasting time and mental energy that should be put into *doing* something.

> *If you want to test your memory, try to recall what you*
> *were worrying about one year ago today.*
> ROTARIAN

Resentments from the past

Probably applies more to stammerers than substance abusers. Stammerers have to endure tremendous disrespect. Disrespect leads to resentment. Resentment leads to stress. Stress makes unfreezing your diaphragm more difficult, takes away from the energy you need to make progress with your speech, and takes away from your ability to concentrate.

What's more, this becomes a present-life pattern where some sign of disrespect will trigger disproportionate resentment. The old 'hashing it over and hashing it over' syndrome. 'What should I have said to that bastard?' 'What will I say when I see him again?'

You must first believe to the bottom of your heart that it is a destructive, stress-causing waste of time and mental energy. Go back and write down in detail every incident you can remember where you wallowed in resentment. **Answer this: Did it help? Was it worth the stress? Was it worth the time? Did it ultimately hurt you?**

Stammering and substance abuse

If you are regularly depending on booze or drugs- to get you through tough speaking situations, you are probably addicted or well on the road. This writer, in his stammering days, has been known to take a few drinks before a difficult situation to be fluent. This writer's heart is irregular because he has also been known to abuse Benzedrine for the same reason.

If you have fallen into the abyss of substance addiction you need to deal with the addiction before attempting to deal with your stammering. Get yourself into a good twelve-step programme. Don't wait until, like most drunks and junkies, you hit bottom. Or maybe you need to hit bottom.

Not addicted to booze and drugs, but perhaps overindulge? If you are trying to reach a solid fluency there are still dangers:

Danger number one: When you are under the influence, you probably speak much too automatic without a smooth diaphragm movement. This is no problem except if there are situations which are causing blocks and trick using. It is especially dangerous if you are regressing.

Danger number two: If you are struggling to reach a satisfactory level or fighting to reverse a regression, you cannot afford to be nursing a hangover. There will be enough days when you are sick or tired from other things.

Pete Sampras probably goes real easy on indulging especially before a tough match. But that's because there are players who can indeed beat him if he is not playing in top form.

To make another point: Pete Sampras with a stinking hangover wouldn't think twice about playing Dave McGuire (but would probably require a lot of money to put up with the boredom). I would still be lucky to win a few points. You, too, can come to the level that every speaking situation will be on the same level as a hungover Sampras versus yours truly.

This programme has seldom or never worked for people who are substance abusers. Probably because whatever is causing them to abuse substances is compelling them to resort to the addictions of stammering, namely tricks and avoidance. Advice? Get into a good twelve-step programme and start controlling your substance addiction before tackling your stammer . . . but, sometimes you can do both at the same time.

Desire for comfort and convenience
Unfortunately, recovery from addiction/stammering requires one to come out of the comfort zone. Which is uncomfortable. Unfortunately, you as a stammerer are dealing with an affliction that is profoundly unreasonable and unfair. You need to declare total war on your stammer with special attention to the tricks and avoidance. War is never fair or reasonable.

Fear of doing something about a serious problem
Really committing oneself to treatment means having to admit that stammering is a problem that requires a major effort to overcome. Some are afraid to face this. They are afraid that the treatment may not work. Or they are afraid it may work: Then they won't have an excuse to not realise their dreams and potential.

Minimising the need for help
Someone whose stammer is once again out of control, who can't climb out of the swamp of avoidance mechanisms must admit that tricks,

laziness, and avoidance are very powerful and he/she needs help from other people. Sometimes we just can't do everything ourselves.

> *Without a struggle,*
> *there can be no progress.*
> FREDERICK DOUGLASS

Friends (?)

Perhaps you are hanging around other stammerers who are not seriously working to eliminate their avoidance mechanisms. Perhaps they are not working at all. You underestimate their overt or, mostly, subliminal messages. Their messages will pop up in a tough speaking situation when you need to practise but aren't feeling like it. Their verbal or non-verbal voices will be in the back of your mind. You will be more likely to lose your concentration, use tricks under pressure, or succumb to laziness when you need to work.

'One common slogan within Twelve Step groups is "Stick with the Winners". Many relapsers do exactly the opposite. They seek out those whose ideas correspond to their own – and set up a "support group" for failure'.

Just as a recovering alcoholic needs to get away from practising alcoholics, a recovering stammerer is well advised to stay away from those other stammerers who are practising avoidance mechanisms. Perhaps when you have recovered you can go and help them but, until then, you need to save yourself.

> *A fool can always find*
> *a greater fool to admire him.*
> *Nicolas Boileau (1636–1711)*
> (L'ART POÉTIQUE)

Or perhaps you have a circle of fluent, so-called friends who have tolerated your company even though they have little or no respect for you: 'Tony the stammerer? Sure, he can come along as long as he doesn't try to say anything'. By struggling to keep these 'friends', you are constantly putting yourself in the 'desire for acceptance versus fear of rejection' approach-avoidance conflict. If

Hold ID... FLE 0629
Hold Until: 11/17/16

IRV Hold Slip
Beyond stammering

you are struggling for fluency, this conflict will lead to the fear-of-stammering conflict.

> *Great spirits have always encountered*
> *violent opposition from mediocre minds.*
> ALBERT EINSTEIN

Face the music. They aren't your real friends. Dump them. Face the prospect of being alone for a while until you find new friends. Or maybe it will be one friend. Or no friends. Having friends is better than the disrespect of being a tag-along. Nothing is worse than being dragged back into uncontrolled stammering.

Or perhaps it is the controlling-type people who need the upper hand and therefore resent you becoming a fluent person. And they'll do things to undermine your recovery. They will increase the time pressure. They'll say things like: 'I liked you better when you stammered.' They'll not confront you when they see you use tricks. They'll help you find excuses not to practise and work. They'll help you avoid situations. They will continue to interrupt and talk over you.

> *No one can make you feel inferior*
> *without your consent.*
> ELEANOR ROOSEVELT

What to do? Take a class and/or read a book on assertiveness training. A controlling friend will either accept the new you on an equal basis or go their own way. Let it go. Don't try to hang on to it.

Aggressiveness

Once your speaking potential is set free, you will have a lot to make up for. Especially if you have had partial assertiveness training. The danger comes when you dump all those built-up resentments on to the wrong person such as your wife or boss. Suddenly you are about to lose your job, and getting nasty letters from your soon-to-be ex-wife's attorney. The stress caused by all this can lead to big blocks and, worse, an excuse to go back to your old ways.

> *How much more grievous*
> *are the consequences of anger*
> *than the causes of it.*
> MARCUS AURELIUS

Relationship change

It is very possible that your stammering dictated your choice of relationships. Your friends/partner very possibly need to control you and don't appreciate having to deal with a whole person now. They might very well put pressure (subtle or otherwise) on you to return to your controllable 'old self'. And the stress of the whole thing will offer you a great excuse to stop the fight for fluency.

> *Never be bullied into silence.*
> *Never allow yourself to be made a victim.*
> *Accept no one's definition of your life;*
> *define yourself.*
> HARVEY FIERSTEIN

Body changes

If you are successful with this method, you will experience a profound personality and probably a physical change. Many have experienced relief from chronic asthma, freedom from common lung infections, lowered blood pressure, more energy, etc.

But you can also experience perhaps heart palpitations from the excitement of a new life. Or you might forget to pause and hyperventilate. Or perhaps you'll forget to eat properly because of all the excitement of the new you.

Unwise decisions

Someone going through such a huge mental, emotional and physical change is in danger of 'going off the deep end'. You might be tempted to break up your marriage, quit your job, go on a buying/spending spree, take out a loan, etc. All this based on your 'new self'.

Don't. Stay cool. No big decisions. Wait until the dust settles. Your 'new self' is going to evolve constantly while you get used to being a normal speaker. This will take over a year. Big decisions based on you as someone who has been fluent for two months will probably not be the same as for someone who has been fluent for two years.

The danger is the stress created by these chaotic decisions might very well become an excuse to stop working (if you need to continue to work), or to fail to respond properly when you hit those surprise chest freezers which I promised earlier.

Experimenting with tricks and avoidance

Tricks and various ways to avoid can be very sneaky. Maybe you'll clean up all your avoidance behaviour, but you let yourself try something new and manage to convince (manipulate) yourself that this new trick is not a trick but something okay to use. The new junk feels great and doesn't (at first) lead to falling back to using the old junk. Again, there's the old dynamic of the honeymoon period. Being clean of tricks and avoidance, like any addiction, makes everything work better for a while. The new trick worked great and didn't lead to uncontrollable stammering. But the honeymoon, as it always does, ends, and the dysfunctional relationship (with avoidance mechanisms) begins followed closely by a return to uncontrolled stammering.

Family problems

On the intensive courses and follow-up of the McGuire Programme, we emphasise the importance of family support and even participation. But sometimes, families can promote a return to uncontrolled stammering and keep someone from getting back on track. Stuff commonly heard that undermines progress: 'Why do you have to speak in this strange way?' 'You sounded so much better before you tried this method!'

Assuming you've tried to explain what you are doing to your family, they still disapprove of this new way you are speaking. They complain about having to wait for your pause, criticise your deliberate dysfluency, and make negative comments about the big costal breath. Or, for married folks, someone, who has worked very hard on his or her speech and experiences significant improvement, becomes in many ways, a different person. Not the same person his or her spouse married. Unless the partner understands the process resulting from this (many times) sudden freedom, she/he could feel threatened. Some can perceive it as 'brainwashing' and take serious steps to undermine the progress.

We can only recommend (strongly) that you seek out a good marriage and/or family counsellor and follow directions.

PART THREE:

Stories from graduates

The Best Medicine
Alan Badmington

I was in intense pain; my back had been causing problems for several days and I could not sleep. We had just returned home from holiday, where the non-supportive bed had been unsympathetic to my medical condition and I was still suffering the consequences.

Wearily, I made my way to the doctor's surgery; I required something to alleviate the extreme discomfort. The usual pills had failed to have the desired effect and I was in desperate need of relief. As I sat in the waiting room, it was rather ironic that I dozed intermittently. My eyelids seemed as though they were implanted with lead; I felt absolutely drained and devoid of any energy.

My usual GP was unavailable, and so I had no alternative but to accept the first appointment offered. The doctor, a youthful female locum, appeared quite attentive as I explained my predicament. But, for some reason, I felt uncomfortable. Could my poor physical condition be affecting my speech?

The supreme confidence I had exuded since joining the McGuire Programme (just three months earlier) had, momentarily, evaporated and I sensed that certain tricks (which had been such a trait of my life-long stutter) were attempting to return. It was extremely disconcerting; I could not understand what was happening.

I succeeded in explaining the circumstances of my medical

problem without too much difficulty, although I was convinced that I may have practised minor word substitution. I had promised myself that avoidance was a thing of the past and . . . now I was succumbing to temptation. The medical practitioner duly handed me the prescription I had sought and I bade farewell. I felt crestfallen and insecure as I left the surgery; my self-esteem and confidence tinged with fragility and doubt.

Upon my return home, I reflected on the occurrence; deeply concerned at my performance. Had the bubble burst? Was this the start of a regressive journey down the slippery slope? Fortunately, I was not permitted to dwell on the matter any further, as I sought the refuge and comfort of my own unyielding mattress. Within seconds I was asleep.

When I eventually surfaced, the painkillers had performed their purpose and I felt surprisingly refreshed. Despite the obvious physical improvement, the memory of the unpleasant experience in the surgery was still uppermost in my mind.

I knew that I could not move forward until I had eradicated the setback I had experienced. In McGuire terminology, it was essential that I practised cancellation. Within minutes, I made a disciplined telephone call to the surgery to arrange another appointment for the following day. Not only that, I insisted on being allocated the same doctor, at a time identical to the original encounter. If I was going to cancel, then I wanted to do it with style. I needed to recreate a similar set of circumstances (albeit twenty-four hours later).

At the appointed hour (9.30 a.m.), I entered the same surgery, where I was greeted by (yes, you've guessed) the same receptionist. I occupied the same seat and waited for the same GP to call my name. She appeared surprised, as I deposited myself in the chair before her, and enquired if there had been any improvement in my back condition.

Resisting time pressure, I paused, secured eye contact and acquainted her with the fact that I was a recovering stutterer. Outlining the purpose of my revisit, I apologised for taking up her valuable time, but stressed the importance of cancellation to my successful recovery.

I believed that my wellbeing was at stake and felt totally justified in enlisting her aid to resolve what I considered to be a genuine health problem. Would she view it in the same light? I fully expected some kind of admonishment (or, at least, a display of displeasure) but, to my amazement, she exhibited considerable interest and developed the discussion further. We spoke for at least twenty-five minutes, while I related my experiences of the McGuire Programme, and acquainted her with some of the contents of the course manual, *Freedom's Road*.

Indeed, when I suggested that I might incur the wrath of her backlog of waiting patients, she made it clear that she would much prefer to continue with our oral exchanges, rather than fulfil her mundane consultations. As we parted, the accommodating medical practitioner confided that I had 'made her day' and requested literature about the Programme. 'Don't hesitate to come back at any time, I'd be delighted to see you,' she added.

I thanked her profusely for her courtesy, patience and understanding, but diplomatically stressed that I hoped my future visits would be few and far between. We laughed, shook hands and I left the surgery feeling ten feet tall. (Indeed, I had grown in stature to such an extent, that I have a distinct recollection of bowing my head slightly in order to negotiate the consulting-room door).

That visit proved invaluable; the original episode had caused me a great deal of consternation, and it was imperative that I replaced it with a positive occurrence. Had I not orchestrated a cancellation, then I have no doubt that the former uncertainty and fear (which preceded my McGuire days) would have festered and multiplied.

Stammering is an interactive, self-perpetuating system of components, which thrives on bad experiences. It is fuelled by the memories of unpleasant speaking difficulties (and associated situations) that have accumulated throughout our lives.

After joining the Programme (and, finally, experiencing the removal of the inhibitive oral shackles), I vowed that I would never again nourish and sustain the debilitating demon that had so adversely controlled my life since childhood. I knew I had to arrange an action replay, without delay, in order to redress the balance, and get back on track.

The 'laws of recovery from stammering' had been contravened on two counts (using tricks and avoidance) and implementation of Law 4 (cancellation) was the best (and only) medicine. The outcome was just what the doctor ordered, allowing me to continue my successful passage to recovery.

Progress
Vikesh Anand

My stuttering came about around the age of twelve. At the time, I was an overt stutterer, very severe. I would bang on desks or stomp my feet on the floor all in efforts to try to get the words out. I slowly learned better tricks to avoid the blocks and by college, I became more of a covert stutterer, meaning I would stutter only in certain situations or certain words. I have always tried to hide my stutter, even fooling myself most times into thin-king I was actually a fluent speaker with occasional stutters. I was never comfortable speaking about the topic because I thought people would view me differently if they knew I stuttered, which most people already knew but I kept telling myself that may be they didn't notice that much. The more I tried to keep this a secret, the more it would backfire on me when it came to stressful situations. I would go through ups and downs in my speech not knowing if the next day would be a good day or bad to speak.

I finally reached my frustration with my speech and looked into helping myself. I was directed to the NSA, National Stuttering Association, by a college friend. The NSA has local chapters through-out the United States and has monthly support meetings. I started going to these meetings towards the end of the summer in 2001. At that time, I was still embarrassed by my stutter that I would lie to my friends about where I was going when the meeting time would come around monthly. So while I was trying to learn more about stuttering and helping myself, I was doing as much harm by hiding it from my family and friends. The meetings were great because I got to meet stutterers from the local area and learn about their experiences as well as how they have dealt with it. Prior to these meetings, I had only met one person who stuttered in my life. These meetings were important because it was the first time I spoke freely about all my experiences, both recently and while growing up, to people who actually understood exactly what I was going through. It is, and will always be, very hard for a fluent person to understand the emotional pain we go threw in life as a stutterer. It is here that I also learned about different programs available to try to help people with their stuttering. I had not attended a therapy session since grade school, again going back to my desire to hide it all my life.

I learned about the McGuire Programme, which was a worldwide programme, but was making its first courses available on the east coast in Washington DC in early 2002. I did not attend the April course as I was still unsure if I wanted to attend any course at all and really did not know if I needed it. Being covert, I could get by in most situations so I thought it wasn't that bad all the time for me. Then in May, I reached a level of frustration with my speech and decided to attend the June course in Washington DC for the McGuire Programme. It was not one particular incident that led me to my decision, but years of holding it in and trying to hide it. The dam had to break sometime, and better it broke sooner than later in my opinion.

I was fairly nervous in attending the course. I did not even tell most of my family or friends prior to going to the programme. I had not attended any form of therapy for my speech since grade school. Also, since stuttering is such a unique problem and different in each individual, I did not know if this would work me just because it had worked for many others. The advantage I did have was that since I did not attend any other programmes, I did not have any bad tricks or routines that I would have to overcome in learning this new programme. The course lasted four days, and I enjoyed every second of it.

For the first time in my life, I was actually acknowledging I was a stutterer, and that self-acceptance alone was such a weight off my shoulders. All my life, I tried to hide my stuttering and here I was doing exactly the opposite. I could, for once, breathe easy and look forward to speaking rather than have the fear of not knowing whether I will stutter or not. The course taught me a lot about life as well. If you fear something, run right through it. After all, what's the worst that can happen. And, only after falling can you truly learn how to walk. Part of the programme involves giving a public speech, in public of course. Our public speech was held on the steps of the Natural Museum of History in Washington DC. Now, to be honest, I really wasn't nervous about the public speaking since I had some many presentations at my former job in front of many groups of people. But the fear struck in when the crowd was being gathered by one of the graduate students, and the announcement was being made that a group of recovering stutterers were going to be speaking. I then realised that I was a recovering stutterer, no way around it. As I spoke about what it was like growing up with the fear and shame of being a stutterer, I realised how huge a step this was for me. Not the public speaking aspect of it, but the fact I was admitting to a group of strangers that I was actually a stutterer. I could not stop the tears flowing from my eyes. They were tears of joy, feelings I had been holding in all my life were being let go. The freedom to speak was finally here. It was an unbelievable feeling to know that I would not lose in this battle. I would not give in any more to the stutter, it would not win.

And, from that moment on, I decided to take advantage of everything life has to offer. I have given in too many times to my stutter but not any more. That is all behind me, and I will not look back. I will only move forward, day by day.

The Long Haul
Brendon Comport

(Brendon's first course was the original pilot group in 1994. He had his share of turbulence, but through hard work managed to become one of the most successful graduates. In 1996 he joined the United States Air Force where he is now a staff sergeant . . . something he could have never done with his previous level of stuttering.)

The purpose of this is to explain why I am successful in my recovery (and hopefully to help shed more light on stuttering therapy as it comes a little further from the dark ages). This is a considerably lengthy subject, and one my phone bill has already sustained enough of over the many ups and downs of this whole thing. Hopefully it will motivate someone to get serious about being fluent.

A good place to start with this subject is what happened to me after April of 1994 when the original United States group met. What happened was what happens to everyone: sweating it out playing tug of war with those tricks and trying to make all the pieces of this method fit together. Even though progress was slow it was a step in the right direction, and I stuck with it. It's reasonable to mess up a few times, and I used my few times up really quickly (may be borrowed a few too). Besides, those were the grass-roots days of this method, now it's a bit clearer what works and what doesn't. To cut right to the chase: the undeniable truth of the thing is: it's only as hard as you make it on yourself, and if you're not serious about it, it's not even worth the effort. The single most important thing I did was stay in frequent contact with Dave and the people in the group worth staying in contact with (the support was worth a few huge phone bills), if I hadn't done that, this letter would never have been written. The techniques we were practising (then called C-P-R-I-E: Concentrate, Pause, Ribs, Image, Eloquence) did start to bring success and fluency, but it wasn't until voluntary stuttering came into the picture. It's a lengthy story, but one worth mentioning.

One of the people I talked to often from that group was Johnny, and somehow during a conversation the subject of voluntary stuttering and Dr Sheehan came up (at the time, voluntary stuttering was only slightly integrated with this method, and I was having little success anyway). To make a long story short, he sent me some first-hand Dr Sheehan material and I worked with it, got a better feel for successful voluntary stuttering (stuttering forward), and with that came a lot of confidence. What better way to kill the fear of stuttering than to stutter intentionally. I got a great boost from this (from the fact that I had taken something I knew little about and in a matter of a few days found some fluency in it), but I knew that (from what David had said about his experiences with Dr Sheehan and from what I had seen in people who had gone through the programme), voluntary stuttering by itself is not enough for most people (because of the incredibly lengthy amount of work necessary).

So I kept working on my diaphragm, kept working on my concentration, kept trying to fight off and weed out the tricks. I kept this up for many months. Until in December of 1994 (and I had been going strong for some time) I had a huge fall. Probably the worst fall ever. I won't go into the gory details, but I will say it was the result of a new speaking situation and two beautiful eyes (blue with large voluptuous pupils) staring back at me (for reasons of professionalism I had better not say any more than that, even though I'm not a professional). Enough to make even someone who doesn't stutter freeze up. Where is he going with this (?), you are probably wondering by now. The point of the story is after eight months of sweat, blood, and hard work I still had a block, and worst of all I handled it with a trick (word avoidance).

This is when I called up Dave and we figured out what happened. I had spent these eight months weeding through the tricks, and getting rid of the obvious ones, and without knowing it letting the strongest one grow and grow until it became the one big hurdle left (at least the only one that has shown itself lately) and the biggest of all. This trick is a trick that everyone who stutters has in common to one degree or another. Even people who don't stutter do this, but the difference is people who stutter need to pay attention to it. The trick I speak of can best be described as 'holding back' or 'back door speaking' (kind of sounds like something you would find in Zen and the art of stuttering recovery, if there was such a book). You won't find this in your Funk and Wagnalls, so I give this definition in the hope that you can further benefit from my experience. Holding back is when you say something quietly without reason to, it is when you slip out a word or a sound at the end of a breath, it is even something like having a beer when you're having trouble with tricks and should be working harder (actions qualify as holding back too). In short, holding back is another form of avoidance. It is also anything less than eloquent direct speech and it is a trick, and tricks always catch up with you. How do you know when you are not avoiding? When you take risks and seek out new and feared speaking situations, when you go out on a limb and say things you might not ordinarily have said. When you make the most out of every speaking situation you can.

To speak or not to speak? That is the question continuously posed to those of us who stutter. To do or not to do? To act or not to act? Go along with it. Stuttering is not just something that happens when you open your mouth, it is a whole personality. If you are going to recover from it, working on the mechanics of your speech is not enough. You have to look at where everything you say comes from. Why you say it is just as important as how you say it. If you feel good about saying something, say it; if you do not feel good about it, take a good look why, because you might be holding back and not even know it. It also pays to look at where the motivation for things you do comes from (that's right, actions are worth attention because they are affected by stuttering, and for that matter anything that you think may be affected by stuttering is worth attention).

Why am I successful in my recovery from stuttering? Because I did not give up or let lame excuses like 'old habits are hard to break' get to me (this old habit may very well be hard to break, but there is no sense in letting it get you down). After that last block I started really paying attention to everything I said in the above paragraphs. Work is what it comes down to, hard work, and getting rid of those tricks. As Dave has said to me many times, 'If you have to jump through a wall of fire you want to do it hard and fast' (analogy no. 10,000 and whatever, but none the less true).

The harder you work and the faster you climb the less painful it will be. Tricks mess up the whole game, and make the person who stutters lose. No recovery from stuttering will work as long as there are tricks. Fortunately, recovery from stuttering is something that feeds itself once it gets going strong. Stuttering is so much work and so stressful that having that energy and a healthy attitude to reinvest somewhere else is very powerful, and once you get it that fluency is worth any amount of work in the world to hang on to. Only time will tell if this method and these techniques work. From my point of view the light at the end of the tunnel is in sight, and if I keep playing my cards right I'll keep getting closer. With the right amount of work I'll bet anyone who stutters can say the same thing.

Recovery
Charlie Caselton
I'm an alcoholic – no, I'm a drunk. I prefer to say 'a drunk' because it keeps me more in touch with where I was. Although alcoholism is a clinical condition, 'alcoholic' sounds way too mature and respectable for a young man like –myself, so let's just stick to 'drunk'. Before I stopped drinking the thought of going for a day without alcohol was impossible, unreasonable, inconceivable and downright unnatural – yet here I am, I haven't had a drink for five years and that feels great. Throughout my recovery from alcoholism I've found the tenets of AA to be closely linked with, and highly applicable to, how I view my ongoing recovery from stammering.

Alcohol always held a particular attraction for me I had learnt from my early teens that alcohol gave me extra confidence and loosened the tongue – what more could any stammerer want? It was the perfect substance: relaxing, intoxicating and FUN. While I consider my stammer as being a contributing factor in my drinking, it wasn't the only reason, but if you're an alcoholic – who needs reasons? I could drink on any excuse, in fact there were no excuses I didn't drink on. However I believe that, stammer or no stammer, I would have become an alcoholic anyway – I'm just grateful I was forced to realise it at 29 rather than 59.

Alcohol wasn't always a problem. It was only my last three years of drinking when I really felt imprisoned, but my stammer has always been a problem to me. It feels like I've forever been a captive held under mouth arrest. From the very first days stammering robbed me of my dignity. Alcohol, if you're a practising alcoholic, also robs you of your dignity, but before it does it will have been a friend; a false friend no doubt, but a friend nevertheless – comforting, soothing, strengthening. My stammer was never a friend. In past speech therapy groups I have been asked to name the benefits of stammering. I could never find any. One possible benefit mentioned by others has been that stammerers use their stammer to stick out from the crowd. This argument always struck me as laughable and rather offensive. There are many other ways of sticking out from the crowd; academic – or any sort of – excellence, sporting prowess, achievement, hell, even fashion sense or some wacky haircut. Perhaps there are stammerers who use their stammer to help them stick out from the crowd, but I suggest that if they are that limp of brain and attitude, and they are using their stammer for this purpose, then perhaps they deserve to stammer.

During my first few months in sobriety I often thought about my stammer and why, if I, a drunk, could stop drinking why couldn't I, a stammerer, stop stammering? After all they are both learned behaviours and as such can be unlearned. They are both things that you do, rather than things that are done to you. Some stammerers may disagree with this last statement but I strongly believe it is true. In both conditions it is easy, and is perhaps part of the initial process, to see yourself as a victim, to throw up your hands in horror and despair and wail 'Why me?' The question 'why me?' is really irrelevant. What is relevant is the belief that we can change. That is the wonderful thing about human beings – our capacity for change, our capacity to improve. As I said at the start, before I stopped drinking I would have thought it way beyond my capability for a day to go by without my taking a drink. It was a concept that was out of this alcoholic's then tenuous grasp on reality. I used to think the same thing about stammering.

Stammerers use many tricks to appear fluent and to maintain fluency once started. They avoid (or substitute) words, sounds and situations, often preferring not to speak altogether to preserve the image of fluency. They speak too fast, they speak too slow, or they begin speaking when the other person hasn't finished. They tap their feet, click their fingers, nod their heads, close their eyes, yawn. They speak too softly, too loudly or without emotion. The variety of tricks used is akin to the variety of drinks drunk. There are literally thousands of them. They can be shaken and stirred into all sorts of cocktails so one might try, say, avoiding a word AND speaking too fast or tapping your feet and nodding your head. Using tricks is a bad and dangerous habit and as with other dangerous habits the tail often ends up wagging the dog. What starts out as a seemingly harmless habit to help you out of trouble becomes an addiction destined to create trouble. On the first morning of Dave McGuire's course four of us were having breakfast at the hotel. There were two Germans who rabbited away fluently for fifteen minutes without a break. Not a single stammer or hesitation did I hear. I marvelled at, and envied, their fluency and seriously wondered if I was on the right course – these people were fluent, what could they be doing here? Sitting with the two seemingly fluent Germans was a silent Scotsman. I sat at the other end of the table. I later learned the two Germans were masters of avoidance. These two could have avoided for Germany on the international stage without fear of embarrassment. They maintained their fluency by adeptly avoiding/ substituting/ changing all words they might have trouble with. Even though they appeared fluent and eloquent they were just as enchained as more visible stammerers. The Scotsman and I both maintained our fluency by not speaking. There is something dreadfully ironic about that, isn't there? – maintaining fluency by AVOIDING speaking.

Avoiding and using tricks is something we would rather not do but nevertheless feel compelled to do. As a practising alcoholic I would wake up every day swearing that today I would not drink, yet a few hours later I would find myself propping up the bar with a pint of Guinness in my hand. Admittedly I would often feel slightly bemused as to how I got to the bar and came to be standing there with a drink in my hand when I had sworn off drink, but that goes to show the power of addiction. How often have stammerers sworn off avoiding/using tricks yet still find themselves, mid-block, wondering how they came to be there? I chose, against my will and my best intentions, to have a drink in the same way that I choose to avoid/use a trick. Even though that part about choosing to use a trick (no matter how involuntary it appeared at the time) always made sense to me, it was difficult to accept. I have found that accepting that fact was crucial in the way I feel about my speech. If you can chose to avoid/use a trick then you can choose not to. You can also choose to stammer. Many people, myself included, have found deliberate dysfluency to be very helpful. Deliberate dysfluency, which I don't do enough of, takes the fear out of speaking because instead of hiding the stammer (the intention of the majority of stammerers) you accentuate it. Deliberate dysfluency puts you back in the driving seat. It works on the principle that by intentionally doing something that you fear, the fear will decrease dramatically. To a stammerer who has never heard of deliberate dysfluency, this technique may appear out of the question. '*What? Show my stammer . . . ? On purpose? – No. No no no no no no no*'. I've found deliberate dysfluency a very effective tool in reducing tension and, somewhat perversely, becoming more desensitised to my stammer.

A major difference between my recovery from stammering and my recovery from alcoholism is that recovering from alcohol is a lot more clear-cut. In AA one is constantly reminded that alcohol is cunning, baffling and powerful. But it is nothing compared to the use of tricks which are all of the above plus sneaky and seductive. You know if you pick up that first drink that you've started drinking again. End of story. Whereas with tricks, often times I wouldn't be aware that I had used one until someone pointed it out to me, or until I started to tape and playback my conversations. So sometimes one isn't even AWARE of the tricks creeping in until afterwards. If a recovering alcoholic picks up a drink he/she will know they've done it. They might be surprised to see the drink in their hand, but they'll know they put it there. They won't have to wait until afterwards to plead ignorance. The one time I've even come remotely near picking up a drink was by mistake. Instead of picking up my glass of ginger ale I picked up my friend's beer. As I tipped the glass back to take a drink my nostrils were assaulted by this vile smell and I quickly put the glass down before I could take a sip. That was a reflex action, an action I am building into my speech pattern to alert myself to the danger of tricks as my nostrils alerted me to the whereabouts of alcohol. Take it from me, once you stop drinking, beer goes from being the amber nectar to resembling nothing more than stale piss.

Alcohol was an easier enemy to fight because its effect was so apparent. I knew that alcohol was making my life totally unmanageable, I knew that I couldn't carry on drinking, so I knew what had to be done. I might have drunk because I had problems but I had more problems because I drank. With my stammer, yes it has certainly added a painful, immensely frustrating element to my life and, yes, I've often felt my life has been stifled, restricted and impeded but we learn to live with it, we learn to cope, we HAVE to cope. In that sense our lives weren't unmanageable, often unbearable perhaps but we could fashion some sort of (dis)order out of our existence. That's the self-image that we've created. Because we rarely see or hear ourselves, our views of ourselves can be softened. It is only on the rare occasions when we see ourselves on video or hear ourselves on tape or spy ourselves in the mirror, mid-block, on the telephone that we realise the extent of the discomfort we must put our listener under. It is then we really see the unmanageability of our lives. We can't manage our voices, we can't manage verbal communication or expression, we can't pretend things are OK and that our stammer doesn't really affect us. That is when the effect of the stammer reappears and we, oftentimes, resolve to get back into speech therapy.

My aim is to duplicate my aversion and strong feelings about my using alcohol onto my using tricks. I was fortunate in that the obsession to drink left me fairly quickly. Not drinking has been relatively easy. It is not something I seriously think about because I know that, for me, alcohol isn't an option. It just isn't an option. I know that to drink again would be a huge step backwards, a step towards some truly horrible feelings. A step to immediate pain, anger and despair. I'd do anything to avoid those feelings and not pick up that first drink. I'd rather be tied naked to a post in a frozen midwinter field and pelted with rotten tomatoes than pick up a drink. If I did drink again the guilt would be overwhelming and that makes it easier not to pick up that first drink. Also the thought of going back into a clinic is aversion therapy in itself.

There are many aspects of AA philosophy and AA sayings that I find I can usefully apply to my recovery from stammering. Having substituted trick for drink, one saying becomes: 'One trick is too many, a million isn't enough.' A basic part of AA life, particularly if you've just stopped drinking, is the requirement to go to meetings. Going to meetings serves many purposes. It stops you drinking for that hour and a half. It keeps you in the company of other recovering alcoholics who, nearly always, have the answers to your questions. It gives you hope because you see how many other, formerly hopeless, alcoholics don't have to drink. One of the great things about AA is the number of meetings available to recovering alcoholics at all times of day wherever you are in the world. While there are, as yet, not enough of Dave's former students to be able to have daily meetings, I regard staying in daily contact with them and Dave, and doing speech practice on the phone as my version of meetings. An AA saying I've heard many times is, 'When you least feel like going to a meeting, that is when you should go'; i.e., when you're finding all sorts of excuses (lazy, tired etc.) not to go to a meeting that is when you should make sure that you go. I feel the same way about my phone/speech practice. When I least feel like getting on the phone, when my excuses crowd in and try to persuade me that there are really many other things I should be doing (like watching TV), THAT is when phone practice/contact with former students is really going to pay off

Another factor I was told about in AA that really helped is that you have to be selfish about your recovery. You have to put your recovery above anyone else's. Look after no. 1. Stick with the winners and don't associate with those alcoholics who are still drinking. It'll only lead to more pain and who needs that? That was an easy thing for me to accept because I was adamant that nothing and no one would negatively affect my recovery from alcoholism. If you stick with the winners some of their magic might rub off on you.

The belief uniting stammerers and alcoholics is the sneaking conviction that their condition keeps them in a place where they know they don't belong. *'If only I wasn't an alcoholic I would ...'* and it's true if only you weren't an alcoholic you would! Since I've stopped drinking I've done things I would never have believed myself capable of doing if I'd been drinking. In my recovery from stammering I'm already doing things I would never have attempted before going on Dave's course. Of course I've set myself much higher goals but I see my recovery from stammering as an ongoing thing. I know I'll get there. I know I'll achieve all my goals. Hey! I have a dream as well – one day we shall all be free. *'Free at last, free at last, hallelujah! Free at last!'*

The Entrepreneur
Bill Windsor, Brisbane Australia

First course: February 2000 I am a graduate from the March course in Brisbane Australia. I have fought my stuttering for forty of my fifty-

three years. Like many fellow stutterers, I gave up on formal education and great opportunities presented to me because of my speech.

At thirteen I began to treat myself. At this stage I could not put
two syllables together. On the advice of an old radio announcer I
began reading to myself in the mirror, using a metronome speaking
in a timed rhythmical manner.

When I blocked I would see that my mouth, tongue, lips were in
the wrong shape so I would stop and start again. By the time I was
sixteen I had obtained reasonable fluency and I was overcoming the
fear of social situations although I never used a telephone until I was
twenty-one. About age seventeen I involved myself with a group
therapy programme run by the Queensland education department.
This group was run by a team of young therapists who used the
methods of the day plus involving us in real social situations, going
to restaurants, shopping and the like but never actually dealing with
the fear and anxiety that we all experienced, particularly as young
adults. However I found a type of voluntary stammer they taught
very useful so I added it to my growing bag of anti stutter tools, but
for me it was back to my reading and mirror treatment.

At nineteen I began my own business because I was too afraid to
apply for a job and employed a secretary to do the phone work. I
was twenty-one before I used a phone. I could tell stutter stories for
hours at this point but at this point I must say that I was overcoming the fear of social and business situations, but I knew there was
something mechanical in my speech that I was not getting a handle
on and that happened by accident twenty years later. In late 1999
while in Memphis Tennessee I had a chance meeting Page
Farnsworth, a speech therapist, who introduced me to the Stuttering Foundation of America. I began to talk to Page about the fear
that stutterers have of the simple act of speaking and how, if you
have never had the problem, you can't begin to know what it is like.
I began to read every bit of information that she gave me. At that
very time I received videos sent to me by my friends at home of the
course in my home town of Brisbane.

In the late 1980s I met a wonderful soprano who changed my life
in many ways, and who pointed out to me that I did not breathe
properly and fully, particularly when I spoke, so when I saw the
videos on the McGuire Programme I immediately flew home and
annoyed the hell out of Rita Sawa until she could fit me into a course.

I was enthusiastic about the course because it was run by stutterers, and developed by stutterers, and not by learned clinicians. In my daily life I have always listened and taken advice from those who have achieved in their field of endeavour and not taken so much advice from the so-called expert professional. I had no idea what the programme entailed, but I knew that I had to learn to breathe.

Somehow it was all starting to come together. I also had no idea that it would be so physically demanding. Having played a lot of sport and being involved in business I appreciated the need for the discipline, which the programme calls for. It is not easy but the results are fantastic. The cloistered environment of the course shows us what we and others with our differing degrees of stammering can achieve with total commitment. I began the last day of my first course crying uncontrollably at five in the morning, thinking of my dear father and how his life would have been so much different if he had had the opportunity that we all had. He stuttered very badly till the day he died. It was also tears of joy for a young lad Adam from Kyogle just near my dad's hometown of Coraki who now had the rest of his life to recover from his stammer and so make a total commitment to his own future not held back by the fear of speaking.

My first course has taught me more than how to defeat my stutter. Resisting time pressure has taught me to listen better, relax more during stressful times and give more considered opinion to what I am about to say. The support group that has followed the course has shown me that I am not the only one who battles with the difficult days. For me, the follow-up and daily contact with my coach has proved invaluable. The sharing of our daily speech problems helps us all. I speak quite a bit to groups and even though it is only a month since my first course people who have known me for a long time can notice a difference in the way I am speaking. For me, I no longer fear the introductions. I will not have to change my wife's name from Carolyne to Ophelia or move the two houses from Wynnum to Manly, if I really want it I have the combination to defeat the stutter. Since the course my speech has had its good and bad days but I remember from when I learned to box that they taught us all the individual aspects and how difficult it was to put that combination together while at the same time avoiding being hit by your opponent. This technique is so much the same, putting the combination together. I'll just keep working on it and doing my best. Travelling as much as I do both in the USA and at home I have met many people with our shared disability from all walks of life. Some like myself believe we have succeeded because of our stutter: it took us out of our comfort zone. While others have withdrawn from the speaking world. But the one thing we all agree on is that we would rather not have it, or the fear of it being in control of our speaking situation. The McGuire Programme gives us the tools and structure to be totally in control of our stammer, to defeat it both in the long and short term.

The New Instructor
Rob Leggatt, London, U.K.

My first course was Liverpool 1998. I did not get on with the McGuire Technique at first. I was still blocking badly on the last day. But I stuck with it, attended the London support group and stayed in close contact with my primary coach, the brilliant Pat Mahon.

Since then I've seen huge improvement in my speech. I chair meetings at work, speak occasionally at Toastmasters with no fear, am a primary coach and certified course instructor. I have my first course to instruct starting 4 May in Cardiff ('May the Fourth Be With You' . . . .)

My recovery has not been smooth. I have relapsed several times. Much of my battle has stemmed from a fixation on my surname. I would estimate that I have done nearly 10,000 contacts on this since my first course. I attack it, kill it, get it to the boring stage. It sometimes comes back. Currently it's dormant. I'm still working on overkill at the boring stage. I am prepared to put in whatever effort is necessary.

On a positive note I can confirm there are no pubs called The Robert Leggatt in Liverpool, Birmingham, Bournemouth, London, Southampton, Swindon or Harrogate. But Sainsbury's do have a fine selection of Leeks, Lettuces. Lemons and Lemonade.

Offloading Baggage
Michael Hay

I'd like to share a story with you about my biggest speaking situation yet which happened this morning. I gave a speech to 600 people at my old school assembly.

Now, although I have done live TV interviews before this was my biggest situation because it was also my biggest cancellation. There was an incredible amount of emotional baggage attached to it.

When I was seventeen, I was a prefect in my school and one of the duties is to give a reading at the morning assembly in front of the whole school. I avoided this completely as it had petrified me and it has been gnawing away at me ever since for the last eight years. When I started the McGuire Programme I knew you were recommended to cancel things and I recognized two main situations that I had avoided which I could go back to cancel: (1) a Bible reading at my church which I had been asked to do, and (2) this reading at my old school assembly. I cancelled the church one quite quickly in my recovery, but for two years now I have been avoiding cancelling the school one. I have made every excuse under the sun as to why I wasn't able to do it.

In Newcastle this September, in the split session on the Sunday morning, Terry Cardwell asked everyone to stand up and give themselves a goal for the coming week. Some said they would use the phone list more, but something told me to use this opportunity for something bigger. I stood up and said I would cancel out my biggest avoidance from my past – my school reading. I don't know if I would have managed this on my own. It shows how powerful the support and motivation from others around you can be. That atmosphere gave me the guts to stand up and make that promise. After I had made that promise in front of everyone there was no going back. No question. No excuses.

I did the reading this morning. It went very well. I got an email from the headmaster later this morning, which said 'I thought the content and delivery of your speech was magnificent'. I have let other McGuire grads hear the speech on my dictaphone and they have said it was great. Although I am on Cloud Number Nine right now, however, I wasn't as excited when I came off the stage. I think there are two reasons for this.

First, although this was an incredibly important speaking situation for me was never nervous about it. I've been incredibly busy this last week and I have never even thought twice about the speech this morning. This is something I would have been dreading for months in advance before the programme, but now I barely thought twice about it. I think this is an incredible thing because it shows I have removed most of the stress I used to associate with speaking. I have the confidence to know I can handle any speaking situation and this is enough for me to just do it. So doing it wasn't as a big a deal as I thought it would be.

Secondly, although my technique was good and I feel my eloquence was high in most of the speech there were still a couple of wobbles at the end. These were really just a lack of preparation (again, because I had been busy and not been dreading the speech I hadn't spent ages preparing) and any slight wobble I had I went back to cancel immediately (that only happened once). Out of 5 mins, 4 minutes and 55 seconds was very good and eloquent, but 5 seconds at the end was a bit bumpy (but still not stammering). Rather than focus on the 4 mins 55 secs of great speech as well as the occasion itself and the self-disclosure in the content of the speech I instead chose to focus on the 5 secs of slight bumpiness at the end. I didn't allow myself to enjoy the moment afterwards.

I feel I am a bit of a perfectionist now with my speech. This in itself says a lot. I never thought as a stammer that I would ever become a perfectionist with my speech! Rather than falling into the fluency trap (I never will – I used deliberate dysfluency at the start and the whole speech was about my recovery) I feel I sometimes fall into the trap of being a proud instructor. I feel that because I am an instructor I should always speak 100 per cent as strong as I do in McGuire courses. I feel that unless my technique is 100 per cent all the time then I've failed. Any small mistake I make I beat myself up about it. After speaking to two people after the event they said that being a good example is not about being, 100 per cent eloquent in every situation (this was my hardest situation yet) but rather in being honest, cancelling, not avoiding, using support etc. I know all this already, but it's sometimes hard to see it yourself. Blinkers etc.

I was probably too hard on myself because this was an incredible situation for me. Listening back to my dictaphone I'm trying to step back and see the bigger picture about what I have achieved. That is why I am now on Cloud Number Nine. The speech did go very very well and I feel fantastic that I have been able to do this after so long. Thank you for the people who helped me see that and also who helped me warm up. George Samios, Heidi Bristow, Alan Wyatt, Terry Cardwell, Stephen Harte, Gareth Gates, Stephen Fletcher and everyone who has been supportive of me doing this in the past couple of weeks. Its this support, which made me motivate myself to do this speech and then also realise what a great thing I had done once I did it. Thank you.

I'm off round the world for a year as of this Saturday, so this is a really great thing to remove some of my old baggage before I go travelling. Its a nightmare having excess baggage in a foreign country, particularly getting on trains.

Cheers for listening!

Story from South Australia
Robert Lucas

I was on the McGuire Programme in January 1999. I was a bad stutterer, who would shy away from every speaking situation, using every trick I could. My whole life was one of avoidances and only making friends through my wife and other friends.

When I first arrived in Sydney I was very nervous and apprehensive about what was going to happen to me on this course. I had tried everything from hypnotherapy to smooth speech, although they seemed to help at the time, they had no long term effect and the let down was they did not have any support afterwards.

When we assembled that Wednesday to do our first day videos, my heart was racing like a runaway train. My turn came and I was adamant that I was going to get my proper name out, not the name I called myself (Bob). I came away from the videoing thinking to myself that I had done a great job in hiding my stutter. When I saw it some time afterwards, I did not realise how severe my stutter was. I still watch it now and then, to enforce within myself, that I never want to be like that again.

Simon Bailey was the course instructor. To me the first day was very intense, where you where shown the new breathing technique and how to wear your belt, this, with the checklist was repeated over and over. We were to learn afterwards that this was the most important part of the course. That night we where encouraged to stand up and say our name and address, a situation I would try to avoid at all costs. I held back from going first and watched in disbelief as other students around stood up and said their name with confidence and without stuttering. Now I couldn't wait to stand up myself and when my time came everything I said was with perfect technique and without that silly stutter, my ears were listening to the words that I had wanted to say for fifty years – MY NAME.

What really opened up my eyes to this wonderful way of speaking, was going out with a coach to do contacts. My coach showed me all the ways to make contacts. Walking down one of the Sydney streets with him (Sam Pring) it suddenly dawned on me this is what it was all about. Facing your fears to talk and approach as many people as you could, from that time onwards all the speaking fear faded away.

The next day we got the introduction to the Harrison workshop that showed us, you could have fun with your speech and then it was our turn to do contacts with the coaches. I was pacing myself with the number of contacts I made. This was easy with the help of my coach. I was talking to people that I would never dream of speaking to. Then came the public speech at Circular Quay, this was the biggest fear I had to face, not that I was frightened of stuttering as I could now control it, but it was the fear of facing a large crowd of people, who were looking at me. Up I got, out came the words, no stuttering, everyone was looking, I made as much eye contact with different people as I could, everything went OK. I got down and felt like a new person. One that was not afraid to speak anywhere, anytime and with out stuttering. Wow! What a feeling.

The rest of the course went by and it was time to go home to Adelaide. My wife picked me up at the airport, and to impress her I took her over to the car rental counter and did a disclosure, looking back at her I saw the joy and tears in her eyes. We both knew that the road to recovery was on the way.

It's been a long road and is still a long road, with lots of little detours that you have to be careful of, because these can lead you to the swamp. Since doing the course, I have learnt more about myself and how people perceived me, than during my whole life.

I have faced all my fears, joined clubs, made speeches at work, done TV interviews, radio interviews, and joined a drama class to gain even more confidence. These days I look forward to facing any challenge handed to me.

Although I still stumble at times I know where I have gone wrong and these days it does not worry me as it used to. I maintain that you must have commitment and without this you will take that detour to the swamp.

By the way I am fifty-four years of age but for the past twenty-two months I have had no fear of speaking.

One of my biggest thrills was to be selected by David McGuire to be a Regional Evaluator.

Another great satisfaction was to be chosen as Team Leader on the Adelaide four-day intensive.

I am in the McGuire Programme to help myself, whilst helping other stutterers.

Losing Fat and Losing Stammering
(gaining a leaner body, and becoming a strong speaker)
Dave McGuire

Compare the dynamics of someone coming into a weight loss programme 100 pounds overweight to someone into a fluency programme with an iceberg full of feared and avoided words and situations. The feelings and thoughts are: 'It's hopeless, I've got too far to go, I can't keep it up, I can't do it.' Well, someone grossly overweight CAN do it . . . others have. Likewise, a grossly severe stammerer who has spent a lifetime in fear and avoidance CAN become a strong speaker in all situations . . . others have done it. Those of you who haven't had a weight problem will have to take my word for it: GETTING RID OF YOUR STAMMERING CAN BE INFINITELY EASIER AND FASTER THAN LOSING FAT.

Spending twelve to fifteen hours a day, including weekends, developing this programme did not leave me the time or motivation to keep exercising or eating right. I had been heavily into tournament tennis for many years in Holland. Long hours of practising and sometimes over three-hour tournament matches on the slow European clay required that my carbohydrate intake be high. I didn't really have to watch what I ate because it was getting worked off. Then I got this darn fluency and the idea to start this darn programme. I stopped playing tennis, but kept eating as if I were going to be playing the French Open in two days.

Bit by bit, my trousers felt tighter. I avoided the bathroom scale. Finally the accursed digital truth machine ran out of battery power and ended up somewhere in the closet. My wife would tell me that I had to watch my weight. My kids would make teasing comments about 'fat daddy'. First thing mother said when she saw a video of me in a BBC talk show was 'My, you've got so BIG!' . . . followed by some suggestions about drinking more water and eating an apple every time I felt those hunger pangs. Dad just asked if I had started playing football again. Then there was that irritating feeling of my inner thighs rubbing together and my upper arms rubbing against the fat deposits under my armpits. But I would ignore all this thinking that I would either accept myself as a fatso or lose the pounds 'someday'.

Well, by the end of 1996 with good coaches handling the programme, my book written, everything seeming to go smoothly, and about two months in December 1996 and early January 1997 with nothing to do before the next course, I figured it was a good time to take a look at my weight and may be do something about it. The old scale no longer worked, so my wife went out and bought another. With hands over my eyes, I got on the new scale, took my hands away, and saw to my horror that I had undeniably become a fatso – 96.5 kilos (15 stone 3 lbs). Great for being a defensive tackle, bad for tennis. Enough was enough. Time to do something.

As usually has happened in my life, a friend sent me a 'new' diet book about a high fat (good God!), low carbohydrate (and no sugar) diet. Without getting too much into the theory, the idea was to simply re-establish the fat burning metabolism cycle.

Of course I was reluctant to start or even read the darn thing for the same reason many persons who stammer don't go into another therapy course after failing a few . . . I knew that there was a huge chance (about 95 per cent) that I would put the weight back on. It had happened several times before. This fact had also discouraged me from going on the usual low-fat diet.

But I made a commitment to not only give this diet a fair chance, but to also change my lifestyle to include more exercise. The weight did indeed come off relatively fast and my energy level rose and stabilized (seems as though I was a bit hyperglycaemic from too much carbs and sugar). And, as long as I paid attention to the diet and exercised regularly, the extra pounds stayed off.

Sure, I've 'relapsed' a few times and had to refocus and recommit to diet and exercise. Just like I've relapsed with my speech and had to refocus and recommit. But each time, both my body slimmed down and toned up, and my fluency returned.

Here are some more connections to stammering:

Stuff that keeps us from losing weight:	Stuff which keep us from losing our stammer:
'I've lost weight before, but regained it (so why try?).'	'I've been fluent before but my stammering came back (so why try?).'
'Almost everyone who diets gains the weight back or more within five years. Losing weight permanently is impossible.'	'Almost everyone who goes through therapy and becomes fluent stammers again within a few months or years. Stammering is incurable.'
'There are many diet programmes, but none really work.'	'There are many stammering programmes, but none really work.'
'When you take weight off fast, it goes back on fast.'	'When you become fluent fast, you lose it fast.'
'I don't like the food you have to eat on a diet and I feel terrible with no energy.'	'I don't like how I sound with these fluency shaping/non-avoidance techniques.'
'I can't get myself to exercise.'	'I can't get myself to practise.'
'I can't keep from eating when I'm under pressure.'	'I can't use the technique when I'm under pressure.'

Response to scepticism about the low carb diet:	Response to those sceptical about the McGuire method:
If you follow directions, you won't regain your weight no matter how many diets you failed.	If you follow directions, you will be able to hold your fluency and it will get stronger.
90 per cent of those who continue with the low carb diet keep the weight off.	75 to 80 per cent of our graduates reach a satisfactory fluency within two years. 50 per cent reach this within a few days.
Just because there are many ineffective other diet programmes available does not mean this programme won't work.	Just because so many other stammering programmes are ineffective, doesn't mean that the McGuire programme is ineffective.

Although you can no longer eat your previous level of carbohydrates and must stay away from sugar, you will find this diet tasty and satisfying.	Costal diaphragm based fluency (even when combined with deliberate dysfluency) is much more acceptable and palatable than the syllabic, prolonged and soft contact speech used in block modification and fluency shaping. It quickly leads to eloquent speech.
The usual excuses for not exercising are laziness, no time, and health problems. Of these the only valid one is health problems although one can get some exercise even when ill.	Unfortunately, practice – especially when still learning the technique and recovering from a relapse, is mandatory. The only valid excuse for not doing so is bad health . . . very bad health.
Sometimes people will forget their diet when under pressure, but they can go right back on it (including exercise) as soon as possible.	Your goal is to develop your powers of concentration, assertiveness, and centering so that you can effectively use this speaking technique under pressure. When you do blow it, then you have to keep trying.

For those of you trying to lose some or all of that stammering, you will lose much of it during intensive courses . . . just like a total fast. Then you will have to maintain a certain diet (no tricks, no avoiding, cancel your mistakes, practice the method, push out your comfort zone) just like I have to watch the carbohydrates and sugar, and keep up the exercise.

Enough! REALLY time to do something!
Frits Boshuijer

My story about the McGuire Programme starts in Hoofddorp, Holland in the spring of 1998. My speech was pretty bad at that time. I was playing tennis (which was pretty bad as well . . .) at a tennis centre in Hoofddorp when I tried to order a Coca-Cola at the bar. When I had my drink (a orange juice, because I couldn't say Coca-Cola or even Cola) and was back at my table, the guy who served me at the bar came to me with a piece of paper. He told me that he had a friend who helped people who stammer. On the piece of paper was the name and phone number of this friend. I accepted it, but thought 'yes . . . sure . . . again one of those people who help you to get rid of your stammer . . .' After a number of speech therapists and therapies, hypnotherapy etc. you get very suspicious about these things.

Normally I throw away these kind of things but I kept this piece of paper for about a year. At this time (early 1999) my speech was really, really bad. I could hardly say two words fluently. I said to myself, now you REALLY have to do something about your speech. It kept me back at work (not making phone calls I should make, not going to meetings etc.), in private (when you don't want to talk your social life is not getting too exciting) and we just had a little baby girl, and I really didn't want to read her bedtime stories stammering. I took the piece of paper I got from the guy at the tennis centre and called the number. The guy who answered the phone, a certain Dave McGuire, was very friendly. He explained what he did, why he did it and how. He invited me over to his place to tell and show some more about this McGuire Programme.

I went over there, still full of suspicion. But somehow this suspicion disappeared very quickly as Dave McGuire was a recovered, or as he said himself recovering stammerer. He sounded very good to me, he showed a video recording of himself from before he started his own programme. I was very impressed by that. The thing I liked most the support after a training and the fact that the training was done by people who used to stammer themselves.

A few weeks later I was on my way to Dublin for my first McGuire training. This was April 1999. Arriving there on the Wednesday before the training I was very nervous, not really knowing what to expect. The Wednesday evening other people from and for the McGuire training started to gather in the hotel. Everybody really was very nice everybody was or had been in the same situation. People who came there for their second, third or even more training, who seemed to speak absolutely fluently, were very enthusiastic and passionate about the programme It was very easy to speak very openly about the problems I had and all stammerers have.

The course itself was fantastic and a revelation for me. And it was a very successful course for me. I did a second and third course quite fast after the first one. And my speech was really good at the time. The hard thing is to maintain this level of fluency. You need to keep working on your speech. After a while I became satisfied with my speech and became lazy. Than I experienced some drop back in my speech and I became less fluent again. But the good thing about his programme is that you can ALWAYS fall back on the support of the other students. Call them and they will help you practise the different aspects of the technique that aren't perfect with you. Now I am a primary coach myself and find it very satisfying to help other people to explore their life with fluency.

Although my speech is not perfect all the time (I am not working hard enough on it), I am able to keep a pretty high level of fluency all the time and a perfect speech whenever I need it. In my work as a project manager, which I'm able to do since I joined the McGuire Programme, speech is absolutely vital, having to talk to people almost all day long. And I thoroughly enjoy it. My fluency is something precious to me . . .

The Welsh Teacher
Kevin Phelps

My name is Kevin Phelps. I live in Wales, UK.

I joined the McGuire Programme in August 1999 attending my first course in Harrogate, North Yorkshire.

For 7 years before joining the programme I had been working as a Primary School Teacher. I coped because for me speaking in front of children, where they don't judge your skills of communication, doesn't carry much fear. Somehow I got by. Although meetings, phone calls and more formal situations e.g. training courses, parent evenings etc. involving adult interaction was at times extremely difficult.

After 5 years I applied for a job as a Deputy Head of a school. Primarily because the job was in Pembrokeshire, Britain's only Coastal National Park, in South West Wales. It is the area I originally came from. A beautiful place that I had to leave to find a job initially but now wanted to move back to raise my family.

I was short listed for interview but stammered so much in the interview that I asked on two occasions if I could leave, eventually I walked out. I was extremely upset and distressed not only because I had seriously embarrassed and humiliated myself but also I knew I'd never be able to pass any future interviews and therefore never be able to move back to Pembrokeshire. It was that experience that prompted me to research 'Stammering and My Stammer' and I eventually discovered the McGuire Programme.

After a few courses and loads of hard work and significant improvement over the control in my speech I felt ready for another interview for a Deputy Headship. One came up in May 2000 and I decided to go for it. The interview involved me giving a presentation for 10 minutes and then being interviewed extremely formally by a panel of 15 people, the full governing body of the school. A nightmare scenario for even any non-stammerer.

However, it was different this time. I was totally educated by the McGuire Programme. I had disclosed in my application form that I was a recovering stammerer, I prepared for the interview by warming up with strong costal breathing (the technique I had learned on the McGuire courses), I telephoned my coaches before the interview and put myself into a very positive mindset. During the interview I used good eye contact, I smiled and paused and all in all gave a strong, confident and thoughtful interview. I just knew it had gone well.

The result was that I was informed soon after, thanks to the McGuire Programme, that the 15 interviewers had voted unanimously for me and the job was mine.

Finally, I was able to move to Pembrokeshire with my wife and children (two boys, Toby and Joe) and build our dream home very close to the Pembrokeshire Coast. Stammering was not going to hold me back anymore.

Since then, I have maintained my contact with the McGuire Programme and have graduated through the programme to become a Telephone Coach, a Course Instructor (I am instructing my third course this year) and a Staff Trainer. This has allowed me great opportunities to further develop my own speaking skills as well as the wonderful work of helping other people out of the misery of out of control stammering.

It is now 2007, nine years since my first course. In this time I have done numerous radio and newspaper interviews, a TV interview, countless lectures, presentations, performed as an after dinner speaker you name it!!!

Just over a year ago I was successful in gaining my first Headship in the teaching profession. Life goes on . . . .

Thanks to the McGuire Programme I really have been given a new life!!!

Kevin Phelps

Ordeal and Resurrection
Glen Masson (Sydney)

I am fifty-four years old and have been stammering for as long as I can remember. I recall early days at school when I would have difficulty during dissertation classes and was constantly laughed at and was the butt of many a joke. Secretly, I dreamed of joining my fellow classmates on the elocution stage but I knew that these were just dreams and that there was no way I would ever be able to achieve that dream.

I then started to think up ways that I could use stammering to my advantage. I soon became aware that I did not have to do all of my homework, particularly that which required oral recitation in class. I only had to stand up and stutter through the first line and the teacher would ask me to sit down. I used this 'pity' of my teachers to get away with many things until a very understanding Christian Brother saw through my ploy and lectured me on the evils of deceit. Nevertheless, although I changed my deceitful ways and started doing all of my homework, my stuttering problem remained.

I recall many a time when my speech was so bad that I would have gladly willed for the ground to open up and swallow me. One of the most embarrassing moments I have ever had was when I attempted to ask a girl, whom I had a huge crush on, to go out with me. I fronted up at her doorstep full of that young bravado spirit, but when her father came to the door the words would not come out. I stuttered and stammered my way trying to ask for her but just could not form the words to make any sense. I could sense that the father was becoming a bit irritated and this only made things worse for me. All I could now think of was to get away, and in my hurry to do so, slipped on the top step, tumbled all the way to the bottom and broke my left arm.

There were other less painful occasions, but the embarrassment was just as acute. Like the time at a French language class I was continually changing my seat in the hope of not being called upon to recite part of the French lesson. Unfortunately, the teacher was awake up to me and waited till the class was almost over before he announced that I would be reciting the whole lesson. Was I the butt of jokes that day!

On completion of school and university it was now time to enter the work-force. Although I had qualified as an accountant, I found it difficult to get a suitable position because of my stammer. At interviews I would freeze up and could not answer basic questions, portraying the image of a simpleton. Eventually, with the aid of some family intervention I got a job as an assistant accountant. The job was fine as long as I did not have to speak to anyone. I would go to any lengths to avoid doing presentations. As I can now appreciate, this was not doing my career much good. But at the age of twenty and being petrified of the spoken word, it did not worry me unduly.

In 1968 at the age of twenty-two, I decided to emigrate to Australia. This was a big step for me. Previously I always had the support of my family, but now I was in a new country, new people, a totally different culture and me not being able to make myself readily understood. However, I made it using the many tricks and avoidances we stammerers are renowned for. It got to the stage where I was quite confident of holding my own among a group of people I was familiar with. Slow progress continued until eventually I reached what I perceived to be a satisfactory level of fluency.

Even though I considered myself to be reasonably fluent, there were numerous situations that I would shy away from. Public speaking was one of them. I am ashamed to admit now, that I could not make a speech at my own wedding. Also with my career, I would restrict my activities so that I would always be in the background – where I would not be called upon to speak and give my views. This aversion to speaking has severely hurt my career and has stopped me from achieving my full potential. Even though I was aware of this, I could not find any way out of my abyss of discontent.

I considered that my lot in life was to live out my days as a stammerer until I saw 'A Current Affair' on Sydney's Channel 9 [Australia]. What I viewed excited me and hope sprung eternal. Here was the opportunity I was looking for – at that very moment I decided to go for it. Well I did my first course in Sydney February 2000. Initially I was confused and wondered if I had made the right decision, because a lot of the coaches were still stuttering. I had not heard of the concept of 'Deliberate dysfluency'. I thought to myself that if this was the case, the course could not be much good. Nevertheless, since I was there I thought I would give it a go, at

Hold ID... FILE: 0629
Hold Until: 10/06/16

IRV Hold Slip
Beyond stammering

least for a couple of days, before making a decision. As it turned out, I completed the course and consider it to be the best decision I have made in my life.

Since completing the course, I have regularly attended the weekly Support Group meetings. These meetings serve to reinforce the techniques learned during the course and are an important part of your recovery. My speech and fluency have now improved to the level where I feel confident enough in doing presentations at work and also social functions. I have since joined my local Toastmaster's group and have already made my first 'Icebreaker Speech'. True, there have been a few falls, but I now know how to get over them.

For me, the McGuire Programme has been an absolute godsend. It has changed my life by giving me the confidence to face challenging situations. For the greater part of my fifty-four years, I have been unable to express my true feelings and thoughts. Dave McGuire has changed that – by giving many others and me the tools to travel down confidently and face any turbulence on the Road to Freedom.

My Experience
Bill Fabian (Sydney)

It's been nearly four years now since I attended my first McGuire Programme course in Sydney in February 1999. I am now able to reflect back on the person I was before that time and who I am now.

In the past I had a couple of situations in which I felt comfortable with my speech. This was particularly true of speech pathology clinics. Outside these few situations I would often experience spasms in my speech that were so severe that I would feel debilitated and totally non-functional. I still have occasional blocks but they are just glitches which are dealt with and then I move on. The uncertainty of falling into a chasm from which there was no escape has gone.

All the joys of life in the past had a shadow cast over them. I found it difficult to really enjoy life, despite the fact that I tried very hard to be happy by intent and accept myself as a person who stutters. It was like an ever-present black cloud hanging over me that just wouldn't go away. My hidden underlying view of life was 'One day I'll be dead and I won't have to suffer this torment any more'. I now feel very content with myself and just have to deal with all those other frustrations that are common to everyone. Life is good.

I was a very heavy drinker in the past. Just about every night I'd polish off a bottle of some alcoholic beverage. Luckily I was not a physically addicted alcoholic but just used it to numb the pain. It was what I used to chill-out and find some peace and contentment for a while. It also seemed to help my speech but I now realise this was an illusion. Now I don't touch a drop. Alcohol causes me to get out of touch with myself and I really find value in being fully self-aware. The savings in not buying alcohol has compensated for the cost of the course many times over.

In the past my wife always made the enquiries when a telephone call had to be made or when making a joint purchase. It's not that I couldn't do it. It was just that there didn't seem to be much point in my going through the struggle when there was an easy way out. I now do most of the talking when we are in joint speaking situations.

I often used 'ah' and 'um' as a crutch in the past. When I was asked for my name it would most times be 'Umb-umb-umb-umBill Arf-arf-arf-arf-arFabian'. I have now eliminated that trick and speak in a much more eloquent style. I had quite a few physical 'helpers' in the past to get my words out. Everything from a leg slap to a knee dip. These tricks looked very undignified and were behaviours that were really out of my control in the heat of the moment. Needless to say, they are all now gone.

In the past I would find myself in situations where it was easier to remain silent in the background rather than draw attention to myself. There really is no place to hide though, and there would always be someone who would say, 'You're very quiet'. My reply would be, 'I've got nothing to say'. This was a lie of course and I now have no problems in making my thoughts known.

I would often break out in sweat and go cherry red in the face when I was caught up in a strenuous blocking episode. Sometimes this would even result in my glasses fogging up in certain climatic conditions. These days I'm calm, cool and collected in most situations. I certainly don't 'sweat it' any more.

At times in the past I had a very small voice. Unconsciously, sometimes I would whisper or just mouth the words I wanted to say. Now I can produce a strong and powerful voice when I need to with very little effort.

Fear and dread would often accompany me when I approached speaking situations. The anticipation was sometimes worse than the act of speaking itself. I now approach speaking situations with enthusiasm and still get a kick out of being able to walk into a shop and ask for what I want in the knowledge that I can do so with clarity.

In the past I would sometimes experience periods of effortless fluency; the so-called 'fluency ride'. I really enjoyed these times but inevitably they never lasted very long and when I came down, I came down hard. I now have consistency in my speech and the uncertainty of not knowing what to expect next has gone.

I tried all the traditional therapies that were available and even though they seemed to alleviate my problems for a while, they never provided a long-term solution. They worked very well in the speech clinic but I could never successfully integrate the methods into my speaking personality. In some ways they even added to the feeling of holding back. Now if I just manage my thoughts, feelings and emotions the rest of the things I do to retain confident, forward-moving speech just fall into place. The thought that I used to muster my resources quickly is 'Stand tall, think tall, talk tall'.

Despite trying to accept myself as a person who stutters in the past, I still felt a degree of shame in my condition. I now have pride in myself irrespective of the condition of my speech. The first time I attended Toastmasters and was asked to introduce myself, I did so by replicating my very worst blocking behaviour, with all the secondaries. I then paused, looked into the eyes of my audience and, with eloquence and confidence, explained what stuttering is and how I was dealing with it. In my time in Toastmasters, three people independently approached me to ask if I could teach them to put more power into their delivery.

All in all, life was pretty tough for me before 1999. The only regret that I have with the McGuire Programme was that it wasn't available five years earlier. This was a pivotal period in my life and when the going got tough I could not get going. This period culminated in a time of career change and opportunity, which will never come again. I blew it and almost ended up having a nervous breakdown in the process. How different things would have been had I gained the skills I have now a few years earlier.

Despite all the success I have experienced in recent years I still consider myself to be a person who stutters or at least one with the potential to stutter. I don't know if that mindset will ever leave me, as I still have forty years of identity to deal with. Perhaps I really don't want to be just a fluent speaker and perhaps being a person who has prevailed over the debilitating condition that stuttering can be is more than enough. I know for sure that the old speaking personality that handicapped me so much in the past is now dead and buried.

I'm always happy to speak to anyone about the McGuire Programme and in fact about anything at all. Please feel free to contact me at <u>willf999@yahoo.com</u> and I'll send you my phone number.

My Journey
Joe O'Donnell
Wishing I was overt

At the age of three, I developed a stammer. And like most kids who developed a stammer at that age, it didn't become a major problem for me until several years later. When I started to build up my vocabulary, I found out that I could substitute easy-to-say words for difficult words. It was about that time that I felt and knew that I was totally different from the other boys of my age, simply because I became very hesitant in delivering my speech and would often say phrases that had no meaning. Apart from that I looked no different from Mickey next door. This led me to become very confused whether I was in a group or by myself After every verbal encounter I would walk away, my eyes fixed on the ground, praying that it would open up and devour me, so that I would never have to face another verbal encounter again, and feel in my chest the confusion on my listener's face. I would end up trying to replay in my mind what I had actually said and more often than not I ended up really hating myself for saying the oddest things, lying and being the coward that I was.

Being a covert stammerer, I never had to roll a word about in my mouth for ten seconds. I didn't have all that facial and body struggle that most people associate with stammerers. All I did was avoid words. No big deal? At that time people didn't know that I stammered, simply because I never stammered in front of them. I would scan ahead for any negative emotional words, open up my in-built dictionary, pick the easiest one to say that would relate to the word that I avoided.

I was disgusted with myself at what I had done but I kept my most sacred secret intact. I knew that they sensed that something was not right with me .They couldn't quite understand the reasoning in my fluent responses and that led them to believe that I was either very, very stupid or had lost the plot completely.

I knew that neither was the case. If only I could make myself struggle like those so very lucky overt stammerers, and then I could prove them wrong. But my lack of courage was much more powerful than my determination to be one of the lucky ones, so I opted for a life of avoidances in order to hang on to my secret.

Out of the frying pan and into the fire

The opportunity arose when I was sixteen years old to be the third generation of O'Donnells to join the highly respected family butcher business. My prayers were answered.

Free at last from the clutches of my sneering peer group. I would never have to sit in classroom and soak up time after time my hidden tears of humiliation. There was a god after all. Then I realised that I had just spent my last ten years or so living my suspended life sentence in an open prison and now the time had come to pay my price to society. Solitary confinement. What seemed like a blunt knife tearing my chest to pieces was now only a thorn in my finger compared to what I was to encounter.

I had to get away from '*How much?*', '*What does that weigh?*', and most of all '*Can you answer the telephone?*' Those three phrases remained with me for years. I wasn't very good at being a butcher. A butcher needs to be friendly, needs to be able to communicate in order to sell his produce, needs to know the hind quarter from the fore quarter and needs to be able to sharpen his knife and keep it sharp. I could do none of the above. Once again I felt that I had failed in life. I would have been quite happy, if circumstances had been different, to get a job that didn't require talking.

But loyalty was such a huge part of me and cowardice was even stronger so I persevered.

Path to Freedom

I finally made the move to make my escape from solitary confinement to enjoying the sound of approaching voices and ringing telephones thanks to Patrick Merrigan, Maree Sweeney and

Victoria Bradshaw. They showed me the path to freedom. They shared with me how they, through hard work, perseverance and initially a little bearable pain, had got rid of their plunging knife and replaced it with the odd thorn in their finger. I hope to reach my destination too, but I need to keep on this road and live by the same rules as all those who have already reached theirs.

Thanks to David McGuire for sharing his programme with us, for all those brave people who helped me and countless others on this journey and for my better half Alice who supported and still supports me 100 per cent of her time. Even if I never reach my destination, the most important thing is that I am enjoying the journey.

The Briefing
Lance Austin

Where I work, Monday Afternoon Briefing is a regular event, and the chance to present a LOT of information in a very LITTLE bit of time; hence, time pressure and pace are often necessary evils. Yesterday, Monday (9 September 2002), I 'pushed that ol' envelope' and delivered my first (FLUENT!) briefing at work, for many, many years. Our 'loving/kind' Director, apparently impressed with my performance two weeks earlier (see below), was determined he wanted to see a REAL presentation from me on one of my REAL work issues; well, I wrote it, gave it, it was good, and I was fluent and in control (!). I even stuck in a big deliberate dysfluency in the middle, and it worked. The TWO-MINUTE briefing (I'm not joking! That's all the time you get!) was the first hurdle, then came the Director's question: that was the hard part! Pause, analyse, clarify, formulate, and don't verbal 'tap dance' too much with the answer, the most important thing. Being first up was also a bit of a nail-biter, but it allowed me to stand there, take my time, start when I wanted to, and be seen as a credible speaker, as well as a credible analyst . . . ironically, yesterday was even harder than the briefing I gave two weeks earlier to a packed house of 200 I had decided to brief on the McGuire Programme Course conducted in July here in Sydney, the outcomes, and what it meant for me, so it amounted to a full-on disclosure to the whole organisation. I had the blessing of my bosses, and the stage was set. I was last out of six people briefing, so I was so afraid that my heart was pounding like . . . a great, big pounding thing! Yet, once I began, I gave the most powerful, in control, and fluent presentation I have ever, ever given. At the end, I also made my recommendations that all of the Defence organisation and all uniformed military members with a stammering problem should be given ample access to the McGuire Programme. Even weeks before, I would have not DARED to step up on that stage (!), to speak to so many powerful people – Colonels, One Star Generals, and other senior Defence civilians of Two-Star rank. The liberated feeling was overwhelming, and the emails of praise that afternoon kept coming. I even cried at home with my wife that evening; I was stunned at how positive the whole experience was . . . and wished that the feeling could have lasted for ever.

Keep your faith, Freedom's Road-Sters, work hard, and keep your faith! My successes I've relayed to you here, still don't stop me blocking with that pretty girl at the bakery, or the nice bloke/guy at my local pizzeria. But remember: When you get a block that seizes up the whole chest, and you feel you can't say the first word you want to, and choose another word, GO BACK to that same person later – not someone else, the SAME PERSON – and do a proper disclo-sure/cancellation. Ask for that thing, you couldn't say before, and ask for it as many times as you feel you need to. That person, if a GOOD person, will think you are so cool, and so brave! It's good for you, it restores your self-respect, and you aren't cheating yourself in the long term at least.

Battling
Patrick Merrigan

It is eighteen weeks since my first course in Glasgow, Sept. 1996. I've had a battle with a feared word 'Sutton' for some time now. I believed I had it licked. I was wrong. Six weeks after Glasgow I took a big fall . . . a crash. I had been invited to say a few words at a social business gathering in October and looked forward to it with a little trepidation. Some time before the evening dinner and after the pageantry, I was told by the golf club President that I wouldn't be speaking. Disappointment but joy, I could relax for the evening . . . my mistake. I turned off my motor (costal breathing) and reverted spontaneously to my former comfortable discom-fort . . . tricks, avoidance etc. During the dinner and after not a few glasses of dry white, the President approached me: 'Paddy, we're starting the speeches soon, you will say a few words?' Oh my God

I'm thinking, what's happening. My heart pounding thinking I can't do it, I'll make a fool of myself before the press and my client. All the old fears came up, confusion and panic. I plucked the courage to go to the president and to my terrible shame, guilt and feeling a total jackass, I lied through my teeth – 'I have to go home urgently, due to a family matter'. I got my assistant to do the excuses for me and disappeared through the side door like a thief in the night. Hating myself for deserting the battle and beating my head above the left ear with my fist, I drove for four hours.

What am I? Where am I going in my life? I can't handle this programme I thought. I really would prefer being dead. I was back on my old suicide road again. I telephoned Dave the following morning, Monday, and after a short period, had me breathing and advised I must cancel what I had done and get back in training.

On Wednesday of that week, I walked into Toastmasters alone. With a feeling that must be similar to going to the guillotine, I requested the person taking the money at the entrance, that I would like the opportunity to speak – this being my first time speaking and that I was a recovering stammerer. I won the table topics award that evening. Had lost a major battle at Tullamore, but countered with a win at Toastmasters. I have won a second award since.

The battle with Sutton was not over though. Wednesday three days ago, at a formal business meeting, I was again anxious about the feared 'SUTTON'. During the meeting it came up in my mouth again. I was playing 'not to lose', instead of 'playing to win'. I was flagellating, feeling I shouldn't be here. My hexagon again plummeted, the enemy the stammering monster was back. I kept my outward composure while inside I was dying. Must get back on the street immediately and to hell with meetings and dinner. It was 9.15 p.m. in Cork.

At about 11 p.m. and having lost count with the number of situations some of them repeated to the same people with the question: 'Excuse me (pause), can you tell me, (pause), where is (pause), ssss . . . su . . . sut Sutton House?' It wasn't getting much better, but no avoidance. I decided I might probably be up all night but the streets were getting quiet and I had met the same policeman twice. I was quite desperate but scrapping and fighting. I was not going home to a sleepless night. I tried to telephone Conor but he was engaged. Went through my checklist. Try one more item. Deep through the chest, it worked instantly, 'the greater the fear the deeper the voice'. I had five or six perfect hits. My hexagon was coming up good. Entered a full pub and with a powerful 'Excuse me please' the whole pub turned to the door. Just about everybody in the pub knew where Sutton House was. Same with the pub next door. One hour earlier, I had great difficulty stuttering out 'Sutton' to a drunk on the street. Celebrated with a Chinese and couple of glasses of dry white. I liked and respected myself and had done my best and I suspect the dour look had left my face. I felt great. Telephoned Robert to tell him he had saved me with 'deep through the chest' but I knew the enemy would be waiting for me the following morning. Called Dave at 6 a.m., thankfully he wasn't in his bath and I dismissed the guilty feeling of his skin becoming prune like during our extended telephone exchange. (One of the things about this programme are the gigantic telephone bills. Believe me, they are your lifeline and mandatory.)

I had choices to make and had arranged meetings away on Friday, Saturday and Sunday. Wasn't much point going to business meetings in my negative hexagon condition. I decided to cancel and reschedule my plans. Back on the street Thursday at 10.30 a.m. in Cork still looking for that elusive and lost Sutton House. Wasn't coming out good, though I was deep through the chest. Damn it, what next. I persevered with 60 situations and headed for a meeting nearby at 2.30 p.m. with people over from the U.K. whom I hadn't met before. I had a forty-five-minute drive and again was searching the CHECKLIST. Fast and Full, Hmmmmm. Let's try a few to myself in the car and on the recorder. Doesn't sound good. Faster and fuller (costal breath). I think I'm pausing at the bottom where the diaphragm has gone from all the way up to all the way down with poor timing and a poor first sound. I stopped the car and drilled for ten minutes. I think I have it, let's find a scalp to take.

Stopped a man in his car, waved him down (little narrow country road) so I could see the reflection in his eye. Expelled residual air, eye contact, good perceptions, fired my now well rehearsed question. Bulls eye. Perfect. Thank you. Let's find a few more scalps and test the remodelled speech. Perfect hit after hit. Went to my meeting and voluntary stammered with the best Caselton 'smooth and slow' I could muster. I found my speech speeding up, must slow down. I was back again and liked myself even better.

Day three, Friday, time to overkill. Hit the street at 10.30 a.m., did another seventy and a little shopping and had fun. Its now 3.15 p.m. and I can honestly say I did my best and boy was it worth the pain. It's great. I forgot to mention that I had already done 200 or so situations on SUTTON before the Dublin course and thought I had it licked. Wrong. Dave says it takes thirty days to break a habit. I think maybe it takes 500–600 or more situations truly to kill your most feared word. But this is assuming you aren't reinforcing the old habit at the same time.

Bad News
There will be times when you may be scared to death and have choices to make. To become a fearless warrior, you must have skirmishes and fight many battles. Each battle makes you a better warrior, though painful it may be. Do not run away, it is much more difficult to return to the battlefield, if at all you return. You have choices, to go back to prison for life or fight the monster and set you free. Only you can do it. The sooner you practise deliberate dysfluency. and expose yourself as a recovering stammerer the shorter the Road to Freedom.

Good News
Battle scarred and victorious, you can hold your head high with the best of them, though you are probably better in speaking terms. You will keep your head, trust yourself develop patience and a greater understanding of yourself and others. You will understand the real meaning of honesty and integrity and yet have an air of the Old Western Cowboys who says little but when they do, everybody listens. Above all you will have dignity, self respect and be able to handle just about anything that comes your way.

Do you suffer from Paradigm Paralysis?
John C. Harrison
(This is the text of a presentation made by the Programme Director of the National Stuttering Project, at the First World Congress on Fluency Disorders. The Congress was sponsored by the International Fluency Association and held in Munich, Germany on August 1–5, 1994)

In the late 1940s a man walked into a laboratory of a major photographic manufacturer in America to demonstrate a new photographic process. But he didn't bring along a camera or film. He brought along a red box with a shiny steel plate, a charging device, a light bulb and a container of black powder. The picture he created was faint but discernible.

'But where's the film?' they asked. 'Where's the developer? Where's the darkroom? Why, that's not really photography!' And so the company passed up an opportunity to acquire the process for electrostatic photography, or xerography . . . a process that has grown into a multi-billion dollar industry.

Why did they pass up such a great opportunity? Because the people who saw the process were suffering from: PARADIGM PARALYSIS.

What is paradigm paralysis? Or more basically, what is a paradigm? As you probably know, a paradigm is a model or a pattern. It's a shared set of assumptions that have to do with how we perceive the world. Paradigms are very helpful because they allow us to develop expectations about what will probably occur based on these assumptions. But when data falls outside our paradigm, we find it hard to see and accept. This is called the PARADIGM EFFECT. And when the paradigm effect is so strong that we are prevented from actually seeing what is under our very noses, we are said to be suffering from paradigm paralysis.

That's where I think many of us have been stuck when it comes to figuring out how to treat stuttering. We rigidly follow a cognitive approach. Or a behavioural approach. Or a psychotherapeutic approach. And our paradigm paralysis causes us to exclude valuable information that doesn't fit our particular model.

But if what I have come to believe about stuttering is true, we already know what we need to know. We just need to draw this information together into a paradigm that integrates these many different approaches. However, to do this, I propose that the professionals need the co-operation and collaboration of the stuttering self-help community.

Why do I say this?

In his book *Paradigms: the Business of Discovering the Future* Joel Barker describes how the person who develops a new paradigm is often an outsider. Someone who really doesn't understand the prevailing paradigm in all its subtleties . . . and sometimes doesn't understand it at all. The PARADIGM SHIFTER, because he or she is not imbued with the prevailing beliefs, is able to see the situation with a fresh eye.

This describes some of us in the stuttering self-help community. Because we did not train as speech-language pathologists, we were not formally programmed in the classic ideas about stuttering. Many of us, of course, did acquire the traditional points of view through involvement in speech therapy. But there are others who have made meaningful discoveries through independent study and observation . . . and just through the process of living.

But are these discoveries worth paying attention to? After all, we're not trained in speech pathology. We don't have Ph.Ds. What can we know that would really be of use to the professional community?

Observing with an open mind

As Eastern philosophers will tell you, one can arrive at major truths simply by observing. I'm reminded of something that Margaret Mead, the anthropologist, wrote some years ago . . . and I'm paraphrasing now. She said – there's a tendency among people in her field to be too quick to relate what they see to what they already know. But to make the real creative breakthroughs, you can't work this way. You need to observe with a blank mind. Without expectations.

You need to sit in the native village and simply observe . . . and watch . . . and observe. At some point you notice that these behaviours over here have something to do with those behaviours over there. Hmmm. What is that relationship? I'm not sure. I think I'll watch some more. And so you watch some more. Now, it may be that you are watching the expected mores and rituals. But maybe not. Maybe it's something completely new.

That's the kind of observing that can lead to a new paradigm. I'll give you a small example of what I'm talking about. I used to buy my petrol at a service station near my home, and every time I drove in, it was my intention to say, 'Fill it up' without either blocking or resorting to any tricks or techniques to avoid blocking. Some days I could do this, and other days, I couldn't. I wondered why. So I began to relate what was going on in my life to my ability to speak.

What I discovered was that on days when I was getting along well with my wife I would have less difficulty in saying 'Fill it up'.

But on days when we weren't getting along, when I was feel angry and resentful and holding back my feelings, I had great difficulty saying the words without resorting to tricks and starter devices, such as 'Yeah, can you fill it up'.

I'm not saying that my stuttering was caused by emotional problems. But I did begin to see some of the subtler ways in which emotions played into the stuttering system. And that was not something I was likely to have explored in quite this way were I involved in traditional speech therapy.

Why not?

It's because speech-language pathologists are generally trained to work within a paradigm that calls for focusing attention only on speech and only those emotions that are closely tied to stressful speaking situations, while those who stammer are not used to looking beyond their stammering for many of their own answers.

Getting Beaten at Tennis (and Speaking) and Why It Ain't No Surprise.
by Allan McGroarty

I was playing tennis the other night against a guy who nearly always kicks my butt. He plays very aggressively and instinctively attacks any weak shots I give him. And, annoyingly, he rarely makes an unforced error. I come to net on his backhand – he passes me. I come to net on his forehand   he passes me. I hit from the back of the court – he out hits me.

We played a series of tie breaks and, as usual, he dominated. However, on one of the tie breaks, I managed to serve aggressively, take risks and dominate play. I aced him. I passed him. I lobbed him. I blew him away, won the tiebreak and he was not pleased. I was a little pleased, but I'm also smart enough to recognise that this incidence of peak performance was a blip. Sure enough, in the next few tie breaks he was back to blowing me away.

Why the blip? Why did my game not hold up for any length of time under the pressure of my relentless opponent? No big mystery – lack of practice. I hadn't put the practice in on the tennis court and I knew it. I was showing up and hoping, against the odds, that my opponent might be a little 'off' his usual form and that I could sneak a few points and possibly a victory. Much better that I practice, practice and practice some more, develop a sound strategy based on my opponent's weaknesses (he has some), and develop some match fitness.

The same applies to recovery from stammering. When I've experienced trouble with my speech, as I have recently, and felt the tendency to hold back, there's nothing mysterious about it. It is in large part due to lack of practice, lack of preparation, lack of strategy. And just as I would be foolish to take comfort from the occasional positive blip in my tennis performance, so too I would be foolish to be pleased that I can now and again 'rise to the occasion' in speaking situations. What's most important is how I am performing across time and in the situations that really matter, and this needs constant evaluation with honesty. Are my successes consistently and significantly outweighing my failures? If yes, then I'm in recovery and moving forward. If the opposite is true, then I'm lapsing back into retreat and an intensive response is required . . .

Reading list

Denis Waitley, *The New Dynamics of Winning* (Gain the mind-set of a champion). London, Nicholas Brealey Publishing, 1994.
Denis talks about all those qualities it takes to accomplish your goals and win the tournament of life. He makes many references to successful athletes and business people.

Peter McWilliams, *Do it! Let's Get Off Our Buts . . .* London, HarperCollins, 2001.
Like the title says, it's time to stop making excuses for failure – stop the 'buts.' He, too, talks about the importance of just getting down to work.

Tim Gallway, *The Inner Game of Tennis*. London, Pan Macmillan, 1986.
This book will give you greater insight into the whys of focal point and imaging the diaphragm. It is one of the best books on getting out of your own way and letting your body (including your speaking mechanism) do what it knows how to do.

Manuel Smith, *When I Say No, I Feel Guilty*. New York, Bantam, 1975.
The original textbook on assertiveness training. Assertiveness is the opposite of holding back and avoidance. Holding back in one part of your life can easily lead to holding back in speaking. Holding hack and avoiding is the psychological core of stammering.

Rogers and McMillin, *Relapse Traps*. New York, Bantam, 1992.
Because of the addictive qualities of tricks and avoidance, a stammerer will relapse for the same reason a substance abuser will relapse. It is important for you to recognise these traps.

Susan Jeffers, *Feel The Fear and Do It Anyway*. London, Random House, 1992.
Great book on dealing with those 'negative tapes' and getting out of your comfort zone. You have to get out of your comfort zone to win the war against stammering.

John Harrison,. *How to Conquer Your Fears of Speaking Before People*, Order it directly from: John Harrison, 3748 22nd Street, San Francisco, Calif. 94114, Phone (415) 647 4700, e-mail: jcharrl234@aol.com
I met John in 1995 at the World Congress on stammering in Sweden. He opened new doors for me personally as well as for my programme. He won the war against his own stammer by taking care of those other places in his life where he was holding back. He did this through hard work . . . doing what he learned from growth workshops and books.

Index